Nurse to Nurse
EVIDENCE-BASED PRACTICE

Nurse to Nurse
EVIDENCE-BASED PRACTICE

June H. Larrabee, PhD, RN
Professor
West Virginia University School of Nursing

Clinical Investigator
West Virginia University Hospitals
Morgantown, West Virginia

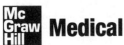

Mc Graw Hill Medical

New York Chicago San Francisco Lisbon London Madrid Mexico City
Milan New Delhi San Juan Seoul Singapore Sydney Toronto

The McGraw·Hill Companies

Nurse to Nurse: Evidence-Based Practice: A Step-by-Step Handbook

1 2 3 4 5 6 7 8 9 0   DOC/DOC   12 11 10 9 8

Set ISBN 978-0-07-149372-7; MHID 0-07-149372-7
Book ISBN 978-0-07-159083-9; MHID 0-07-159083-8
PDA card ISBN 978-0-07-159084-6; MHID 0-07-159084-6

This book was set in Berkeley Book by International Typesetting and Composition.
The editors were Quincy McDonald and Karen Davis.
The production supervisor was Catherine H. Saggese.
Production management was provided by Preeti Longia Sinha, International Typesetting and Composition.
The book designer was Eve Siegel.
The cover designer was David Dell'Accio.
The index was prepared by Susan Hunter.
RR Donnelley was printer and binder.

This book is printed on acid-free paper.

Library of Congress Cataloging-in-Publication Data

Larrabee, June H.
    Nurse to nurse. Evidence-based practice / June H. Larrabee.
        p. ; cm.
    Includes bibliographical references and index.
    ISBN-13: 978-0-07-149372-7 (pbk.)
    ISBN-10: 0-07-149372-7 (pbk.)
    1. Evidence-based nursing.   I. Title.   II. Title: Evidence-based practice.
    [DNLM: 1. Nursing Care—methods—Handbooks.   2. Evidence-Based
Medicine—methods—Handbooks.   3. Models, Nursing—Handbooks.
    WY 49 L333n   2009]
    RT84.5.L37   2009
    610.73—dc22
                                                    2008025680

This book is dedicated to all nurses
who ever wanted to make a difference
and to their patients—past, present, and future.

This book is also dedicated to the loving memory of my daughter,
Lauralee Kathryn (Kathy) Larrabee.

Contents

Preface

Evidence-based practice is rapidly becoming a goal of many nurses and nurse leaders. Achieving evidence-based practice requires making it a strategic goal of the organization and following a systematic process. A number of evidence-based practice models exist in the literature and have been successfully applied by teams of nurses to make evidence-based practice changes. Successful application of these models requires nurses to acquire some knowledge and skills that they did not previously possess.

This book is designed to help nurses begin to acquire the new knowledge and skills needed to participate in and, with experience, lead evidence-based practice projects. The purposes of this book are to describe evidence-based practice and how to apply the steps in the Model for Evidence-Based Practice Change. This model is a revised and updated version of the Model for Change to Evidence-Based Practice.*

The original model was based on theoretical and empirical literature about change theory, research utilization, and evidence-based practice and reflected the authors' independent experiences in leading nurses in research utilization in different acute-care hospitals. The authors of the original model also collaborated in testing the Model for Change to Evidence-Based Practice. Since its publication, the original model has been applied by many teams of nurses and practitioners in other disciplines in diverse settings to make evidence-based practice changes. The changes reflected in the revised Model for Evidence-Based Practice Change are based on the author's experience in mentoring nurses in the use of the Model for Change to Evidence-Based Practice since it was published in 1999 and the experiences of nurses who have applied the model. The revised model also reflects the author's experience with leading nursing quality improvement programs and incorporates concepts from continuous quality improvement.

*Rosswurm MA, Larrabee JH. A model for change to evidence-based practice. *Image J Nurs Sch.* 1999;31(4):317–322.

The book is intended as a handbook for direct-care nurses in any health-care setting as they collaborate among themselves and with representatives of other disciplines in making systematic evidence-based practice changes. The book will also be useful to advanced practice nursing students and advanced practice nurses as they develop skills in leading and mentoring nurses in evidence-based practice change. It includes background information on the pursuit of excellence in health care, the evidence-based practice movement, a description of the Model for Evidence-Based Practice Change, specific details about activities in each step of the model, sample tools that may be used during specific steps, and references to electronic and print resources. The discussion of applying the steps in the model integrates evidence from translation science about effective strategies for change, the use of tools from continuous quality improvement, and working in teams. Cases and examples illustrate the concepts discussed and the steps in the model. To provide a progressively developed case illustrating the six steps in the model, a case describing a fictitious or fabricated chronic heart failure evidence-based practice project is presented in the chapters describing the steps.

Although participating in evidence-based practice change requires additional learning for many nurses, it provides them with the opportunity to have control of their practice, something that many nurses highly prize. Making successful evidence-based practice changes is personally rewarding and, for many nurses, generates enthusiasm for future opportunities to improve practice and patient outcomes.

Acknowledgments

Writing a book while continuing your usual work and personal responsibilities is no small feat. For that reason, I first acknowledge those who emotionally supported and encouraged me during this process. This book would not have been written were it not for the encouragement and support of my best friend and husband, James Larrabee. I am deeply grateful for the encouragement of Dorothy Oakes, Georgia Narsavage, E. Jane Martin, and Susan McCrone. As always, I am grateful for the love and prayers from my mother, Barbara F. Hansen, and my sister, Ellen Hansen. The love of many other family members sustained me during "crunch" times, including that of my other siblings: Stephen A. Miller (deceased), Arie Miller, Kathryn Cowan, and Keith Hansen. Many thanks to my husband's dear cousins, who have been so supportive: Barbara Ann Gillis, Kathe McKnight, and Debbie Walker. Finally, I am grateful to my late father, Glenn Arthur Hansen, for many reasons, including his saying to me when I was a senior in high school: "You can do anything you decide you want to do." I believed him. It made all the difference in the world.

Second, I acknowledge those who gave me opportunities to develop expertise in the knowledge and skills that eventually prepared me to write this book. Most notably, those persons include Norma Mash, Lynn Smith, Joan Salmon, Michael A. Carter, Veronica Engle, Marie Ray Knight, E. Jane Martin, Michelle A. Janney, Dorothy W. Oakes, and Mary Ann Rosswurm. In Mary Ann, I had a special colleague because of our mutual interest in leading programs to help nurses improve the quality of care through using the best available evidence. I acknowledge the nurses at West Virginia University Hospitals who have collaborated with me since 1998 in leading our nursing research program to success: Mary Lynne Withrow, Mary F. Fanning, Jackie Sions, Christine Daniels, and Andrea Ferretti. Many nurses collaborated among themselves and with people from other disciplines to achieve evidence-based practice changes for many aspects of care. They are gratified and proud of the fact that their work helped West Virginia University Hospitals become Magnet certified in 2005. I am proud of their accomplishments, and I know that they can continue to be successful, as can many other nurses elsewhere who make the journey to evidence-based practice. We all owe it to our patients and ourselves.

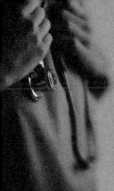

Chapter 1

THE JOURNEY TO EXCELLENCE IN PATIENT CARE

EXCELLENCE AS A GOAL IN NURSING CARE

Ethical Considerations

Nurses have pursued excellence in health care since Florence Nightingale began studying patient outcomes of care processes in the 1860s.[1,2] Subsequently, health-care professionals have launched many initiatives to improve the quality of care. Advocacy for evidence-based practice (EBP) is a fairly recent initiative with demonstrated effectiveness in improving the quality of care and patient outcomes.

A number of authors have attempted to define quality of care. The Institute of Medicine's definition is: "The degree to which health services for individuals and populations increase the likelihood of desired health outcomes and are consistent with current professional knowledge."[3] A definition of quality synthesized from ethical and economic perspectives follows:

> Quality is the presence of socially acceptable, desired attributes within the multifaceted holistic experience of being and doing and quality encompasses, at least, the four interrelated concepts: value, beneficence, prudence, and justice. Value is defined as: (a) something intrinsically desirable; (b) relative worth, utility, or importance; and (c) a fair return in goods, services, or money for something exchanged. Beneficence is defined as actual or potential capability for (a) producing good and (b) promoting well-being. Beneficence encompasses harmlessness. Well-being is of value to individuals, groups, and society, but Aristotle viewed general welfare of society as preeminent to the well-being of individuals. Prudence is defined as: (a) good judgment in setting realistic goals and (b) good judgment and skill in using personal resources to achieve goals. Justice is defined as fairness, which has these two components: (a) distributive justice, using common resources proportionately to the individual's contribution to those resources and (b) corrective justice, correcting an injustice by finding the mean between the extremes of profit and loss.[4, p. 356]

This definition of quality integrates the ethical principles of value, beneficence, prudence, and justice, and, when applied to health care, infers that the pursuit of high-quality or excellent health care is an ethical obligation of nurses and other health-care providers. The ethical principles of beneficence and justice are the basis of the American Nurses Association Code of Ethics for Nurses, along with the ethical principles of respect, nonmalfeasance, fidelity, and autonomy.[5] Nurses are accountable to the public for fulfilling their ethical responsibilities for benefiting care recipients and doing no harm. The most recent version of the Code of Ethics specifies that the code applies "to all nurses in all roles and settings."[5, p. 6] Because of these ethical obligations, direct-care nurses, nurse leaders, and nursing professional organizations have goals for quality of care. Still, the achievement of high-quality health care and the best patient outcomes for many health issues is delayed by lengthy intervals between the dissemination of research findings and the adoption of changes in practice.[6–9] Deliberate, conscientious efforts are required to successfully pursue EBP.

Goal of Direct-Care Nurses

Direct-care nurses have the personal goal of providing the best care to their patients with each patient encounter. When nurses perceive that they can provide the best care to their patients and have control of their practice, they experience job satisfaction and are likely to intend to remain with their employer.[10,11] When nurses perceive that they cannot provide the best care to their patients and that problems in the work environment are the reason, they experience job dissatisfaction and are more likely to intend to seek a different work setting. Turnover of RNs compromises the work environment by the loss of experienced nurses and by adding to the workload of the remaining nurses.

Goal of Nursing Division Leaders

Nurse leaders also have the goal of ensuring that patients receive the best care because it is the right thing to do. Unlike direct-care nurses, nurse leaders have fiscal accountability as a major responsibility of their role. They must make judgments about expenditures based on the best information available to them. There is good evidence that successful EBP change can improve patient outcomes. There is also good evidence that the leadership, commitment, and support of top management contribute to successful EBP change.[12] For these reasons and to encourage nurse retention, nurse leaders should be highly motivated to provide the necessary support to allow nurses to pursue EBP, providing them with a means for having some control of their practice.

Goal of Nursing Professional Organizations

Professional nursing organizations were created over the past 100+ years for the purpose of setting standards of excellence for education and practice for the discipline of nursing as a whole or for specialties within nursing. The oldest organizations include the National League for Nursing (NLN)[13] and the American Nurses Association (ANA).[14] One goal of the NLN is to lead in setting standards of excellence in nursing education. The ANA web site has numerous standards for excellence in nursing practice. Regarding standards of practice, one definition of standards is "authoritative statements that describe the level of care or performance common to the profession of nursing by which the quality of nursing practice can be judged."[15] A subsidiary of ANA, the American Nurses Credentialing Center (ANCC), developed the Magnet Recognition Program to recognize health-care organizations that provide excellent nursing care.[16] The forces of magnetism underpinning that program include the pursuit of continuous quality improvement (CQI) and EBP. Magnet recognition has become a highly desired goal of many nurse leaders in the United States as a means of nurse retention and of validating excellence in patient care.

The Oncology Nursing Society (ONS) is an example of a specialty nursing organization. Its mission is to promote excellence in oncology nursing and high-quality cancer care. Among the resources on the ONS web site is a web page entitled "Evidence Based Practice Resource Area," with links to educational information about EBP and reviews of evidence.[17] Another example of a specialty nursing organization is the American Association of Critical-Care Nurses (AACN), whose mission is to provide nurses with expert knowledge so that they can fulfill their obligations to patients and their families for excellent care.[18] A number of practice standards are available at the

AACN web site. There are many specialty nursing organizations with similar missions and resources for their specialty groups.

From this brief discussion, it is clear that all nurses have goals related to quality of care. There are system-, organizational-, and individual-level factors that influence the ability to give excellent care.

FACTORS INFLUENCING THE ABILITY TO GIVE EXCELLENT CARE

System Level

At the macro level of the U.S. health-care system, there have been a number of progressive initiatives intended to improve the quality and safety of care. Those quality initiatives have been either voluntary or mandatory (legislated). They have focused on

- Licensure of practitioners
- Education program accreditation
- Health-care organization accreditation
- Policy initiatives
- Continuous quality improvement
- Research utilization
- Evidence-based practice

Licensure of Practitioners

The intent of licensure was to establish the qualifications of practitioners and to safeguard the public.

- 1903: North Carolina was the first state to enact a registration law.
- 1938: New York was the first state to
  — define scope of practice and
  — require mandatory licensure.

All state governments followed suit and established boards of nursing whose mission is to protect the health of the public by ensuring the safe practice of nursing. Each state board sets standards for and approves schools to educate nursing students to be eligible to take the National Council Licensure Examination. The state board monitors licensees' compliance with state laws and takes action against the licenses of nurses engaging in unsafe practices.[19]

Education Program Accreditation

Voluntary accreditation of schools of nursing was initiated by the American Society of Superintendents of Training Schools of Nurses, which was founded in 1893 to establish and maintain standards for schools of nursing.

* 1917: Name changed to the National League of Nursing Education.

  — Published the first set of curricular standards.

* 1952: National League of Nursing Education combined with two other organizations to become the National League for Nursing (NLN).

* 1952: U.S. Department of Education first recognized NLN as an accrediting organization.

In 1969, the American Association of Colleges of Nursing was founded to

* "establish quality standards for bachelor's and graduate-degree nursing education,

* assist deans and directors to implement those standards, and

* influence the nursing profession to improve health care."[20]

The AACN developed the Commission on Collegiate Nursing Education (CCNE), which is an accrediting agency whose aim is to ensure "the quality and integrity of baccalaureate and graduate education programs preparing effective nurses."[21] The CCNE began conducting accreditation reviews in 1998.

Health-Care Organization Accreditation

Voluntary health-care organization accreditation originated as a result of recommendations by Ernest Codman, MD

(1869–1940), a surgeon in Boston in the early 1900s.[22] He is recognized as the founder of outcomes management.

- 1910: Advocated an "end result system of hospital standardization" involving
  — performance measurement of outcomes and publication of outcomes to help patients make choices about physicians and hospitals.
- 1913: Cofounded the American College of Surgeons (ACS) and its Hospital Standardization Program.
- 1917: ACS published its first Minimum Standard for Hospitals (1 page).
- 1926: ACS published its first standards manual (18 pages).
- 1951: Joint Commission on Accreditation of Hospitals (later the Joint Commission on Accreditation of Healthcare Organizations) was created by the union of
  — ACS
  — American College of Physicians
  — Canadian Medical Association and
  — American Hospital Association.
- 1965: Congress passed Social Security Amendments requiring certification by an organization such as the Joint Commission on Accreditation of Healthcare Organizations (the Joint Commission) to receive reimbursement for care given to Medicare and Medicaid beneficiaries.
- 1987: The Joint Commission initiated its Agenda for Change.
  — Put emphasis on actual organization performance (outcomes).
  — Was philosophically based on principles of CQI.
- 1992: The Joint Commission began requiring evidence of performance improvement.
- 1997: The Joint Commission initiated ORYX: The Next Evolution in Accreditation.
  — Placed emphasis on *outcomes* and other performance measures.

- 2000: The Joint Commission initiated random, unannounced *follow-up* survey visits.
- 2003: The Joint Commission established a 30-member Nursing Advisory Council to address recommendations from the Institute of Medicine
  — Health Care at the Crossroads: Strategies for Addressing the Evolving Nursing Crisis.
- 2007: The organization shortened its name from the Joint Commission on Accreditation of Healthcare Organizations to the Joint Commission.
- 2007: The Joint Commission initiated the conduct of unannounced *initial* survey visits in hospitals and critical access hospitals.

In addition to hospitals, the Joint Commission accredits ambulatory care, assisted living, behavioral health care, home care, laboratory service, long-term care, networks, and office-based surgery organizations. Also, the Joint Commission offers certification in health-care staffing services, transplant centers, and disease-specific care.[23] Disease-specific care certifications include

- Chronic kidney disease
- Chronic obstructive pulmonary disease
- Inpatient diabetes
- Lung-volume reduction surgery
- Primary stroke center
- Ventricular assist device

Policy Initiatives

In addition to Congress requiring accreditation by an authorized accrediting organization to receive reimbursement for care given to Medicare and Medicaid beneficiaries, there have been many policy initiatives aimed at improving the quality of care. Discussion of those is beyond the scope of this book. One will be discussed as an example: the Institute of Medicine's Quality of Health Care in America project.[24]

- Institute of Medicine
  — A nonprofit organization chartered in 1970 as a component of the National Academy of Sciences.
  — Mission: to serve as an adviser to the nation to improve health by
    ▪ providing unbiased, evidence-based, and authoritative information and advice concerning health and science policy to
    ○ policy makers
    ○ professionals
    ○ leaders in every sector of society, and
    ○ the public at large.
- Quality of Health Care in America project
  — Initiated in June 1998.
  — Launched to address "widespread and persistent, systemic shortcomings in quality" in the health-care system in America.
  — Charged with developing a strategy that will result in a threshold improvement in quality by 2008.
- IOM's Quality of Health Care in America project reports:
  — To Err Is Human: Building a Safer Health System (1999)
  — Crossing the Quality Chasm: A New Health System for the 21st Century (2001).
  — Preventing Medication Errors: Quality Chasm Series (2006).
  — Improving the Quality of Health Care for Mental and Substance-Use Conditions: Quality Chasm Series (2005).
  — Keeping Patients Safe: Transforming the Work Environment of Nurses (2004).

All of these reports have identified serious problems with the quality of care in the U.S. health-care system. They have also provided recommendations for policy makers, health-care organization leaders, and providers. Central to the recommendations is the pursuit of EBP and CQI.

Quality Improvement

Quality improvement (QI) is "a planned approach to transform organizations by evaluating and improving systems to achieve better outcomes."[25, p. 10] The concept and process of statistical quality control, which evolved from the 1920s on, were antecedents to QI as it is known today. Statistical quality control aims at reducing variability in processes and their outcomes, and uses statistical process control techniques to track, trend, and analyze data and to identify opportunities for improving processes.

Statistical quality control

Statistical quality control was originated by Walter Shewhart, a physicist and statistician at Bell Telephone Laboratories, who studied the elements of a process that resulted in the production of faulty parts. He developed the statistical process control chart.

- Statistical quality control involves collecting data, plotting means on a run chart, and calculating the combined mean and standard deviation.
- A process was considered to be "in control" if subsequent means were within three standard deviations of the combined mean.

Shewhart also developed the Cycle for Learning and Improvement, containing four continuous steps: Plan, Do, Study, and Act.

Continuous quality improvement

W. Edwards Deming and Joseph M. Juran, who both studied with Shewhart, are the best-known leaders in CQI. Individually, they further developed their own thinking about CQI and formed their own consulting businesses, providing CQI consulting to manufacturers, a variety of businesses, and governments for many years. After the end of World War II, they both taught CQI principles to members of the Union of Japanese Scientists and Engineers and are credited with reviving the Japanese economy. Both Deming and Juran developed the philosophy that most errors or poor outcomes are related to the work environment, not the workers' skills.

In health care, during the 1960s to 1980s, efforts to improve care focused on quality assessment and quality assurance. Quality assurance processes included assessing indicators of care based on standards and counseling the person or persons thought to be responsible for failure to meet standards. Quality assessment activities were largely guided by Avedis Donabedian's evaluation model, which proposed that structure influences process and processes influence outcomes.[26,27] Structure, process, and outcomes are also factors that Shewhart evaluated when studying the manufacturing process for causes of the production of faulty parts. However, the adoption of CQI by health-care organizations did not occur until the Joint Commission announced its Agenda for Change in 1987 and, subsequently, revised the standards manual to require performance improvement through the use of CQI. Since then, health-care organization leaders have provided support for nurses and other providers and employees working in teams to study and resolve systems problems. That teamwork experience will benefit some persons as they pursue EBP.

Research Utilization

Because of lack of familiarity, nurses can be confused about the difference between research, CQI, and research utilization (RU). Research is scientifically rigorous, systematic inquiry to build a knowledge base. Research answers questions about *efficacy,* or "What are the right things to do?" Continuous quality improvement answers questions about effectiveness, or "Are the right things being done right?" Research utilization is deliberately using research to improve clinical practice, integrating "specific processes in transforming knowledge into practice activities, creating a climate for practice change, planning for and implementing the change, and evaluating the effects of the practice change."[28, p. xiv] Nurses began using RU more than 30 years ago to improve the quality of care.[28–31] Research utilization is only one aspect of EBP because there are other sources of evidence in addition to research. Research utilization has been guided by a number of process models[32–37] that have helped teams of nurses and persons in other disciplines improve care.

Evidence-Based Practice

Evidence-based practice is the simultaneous use of "individual clinical expertise" and "the best available external clinical evidence from systematic research" to guide clinical decision making, while considering the patient's values.[38, p. 17] A number of process models have been developed, and their application has resulted in EBP for individual patients and groups of patients.[39–47] The model described in this book is a revised version of the Model for Change to Evidence-Based Practice.[40] The revisions were warranted by the author's observations and experiences in serving as research teacher and mentor at West Virginia University Hospitals and by newer knowledge about effective strategies for EBP change.

Organization Level

Top management commitment, advocacy, and support for the new standard of care have been effective in contributing to successful EBP change.[12,48–50] The support that is needed includes dedicated time and resources for stakeholders to participate in the innovation adoption process.[51–53] The chief nurse executive (CNE) must include EBP in the strategic plan for the nursing division and use multiple means to communicate this expectation to all nurses in the division.[54] The CNE must provide means for directors and managers to place a high value on EBP because they will be instrumental in supporting the work of EBP teams. Evidence indicates that nurse leaders' role modeling of EBP and communicating the value of research enhances EBP change by nurses.[55] The CNE and the nursing administrative council must develop the organizational infrastructure necessary to support the pursuit of EBP. They must identify and provide the human and material resources needed to facilitate an EBP program.

Human resources include a research mentor, educational sessions on EBP for nurses, time out of staffing for nurses to participate in EBP projects, decision support personnel, and staff support for EBP teams. Education and mentoring about EBP is especially important because participating effectively on a team requires some additional knowledge and skills that most nurses do not have.[56] Material resources include access to computers and electronic bibliographic databases, travel drives or floppy disks, copy machines, paper, and filing supplies.

Nurse leaders should consider developing, adapting, or adopting a log for quantifying organizational support for EBP. Nurse leaders and direct-care nurses at West Virginia University Hospitals have developed and published such a tool.[57] Each EBP team member keeps track of the hours spent in various activities and of resource expenditures. Time expense is calculated by multiplying the number of hours listed by the average hourly salary for the position listed on the form. The data are summarized quarterly and reported annually to the Nursing Research Council. The data in the form are used in budgetary planning for the following year. Also, the annual summaries document organizational support for EBP.

Individual Level

Nurses have a goal of giving the best care to each patient. Many nurses are willing to be involved in activities that lead to EBP change. However, not all nurses perceive that they have a responsibility to be involved in participating in such activities.[58] Some nurses will decline the opportunity to participate on an EBP team for a variety of reasons, including lack of interest, concern about its interfering with their personal life, and feeling overcommitted. Regardless, nurses can do many things to stay prepared to provide high-quality, safe patient care, including

- Attending continuing education sessions
- Taking continuing education modules
- Reading current clinical journal articles and discussing them with peers
- Participating on the Practice, Quality Improvement (QI), or Education Council

- Maintaining balance in their personal life:
    — Personal relationships
    — Adequate nutrition, exercise, and sleep

To pursue EBP, direct-care nurses can do a number of things, including

- Reading research articles and discussing them with peers or with a research mentor
- Attending educational sessions on "how to do" EBP
- Proposing to nurse leaders that the unit or department charter an EBP team
- Volunteering to serve on an EBP team
- Reading a basic-level research textbook
- Taking a course or a refresher course about research
- Volunteering to be a change champion or data collector for an EBP team
- Participating in giving feedback to an EBP team during the pilot of a new practice

The extent to which nurses choose to be involved in EBP change will depend, in part, on their

- Attitudes about the benefits of using research to improve care
- Knowledge about research
- Skills in locating and critically appraising research
- Perception of the value the nurse leader places on research
- Perception of the nurse leader's support for pursuing EBP
- Perception of the adequacy of resources to support pursuing EBP

The following chapters present the revised Model for Change to Evidence-Based Practice and the steps in the model. The chapters on the steps explain how to apply the model. Explanations are accompanied by a number of forms and examples of completed forms. There are also case examples to illustrate the application of the model. To allow for a progressive example throughout the chapters, the author created a fabricated case focused on chronic heart failure.

REFERENCES

1. Chance KS. The quest for quality: An exploration of attempts to define and measure quality nursing care. *Image (IN)*. Jun 1980;12(2):41–45.
2. Mitchell K. The synergistic relationship between ethics and quality improvement: Thriving in managed care. *J Nurs Care Qual*. 1996;11(1):9–21.
3. Lohr KN, ed. *Institute of Medicine. Medicare: A Strategy for Quality Assurance*. Washington, DC: National Academy Press; 1990.
4. Larrabee JH. Emerging model of quality. *Image J Nurs Sch*. 1996;28(4):353–358.
5. Hook KG, White GB. ANA Code of Ethics for Nurses with Interpretive Statements. http://nursingworld.org/mods/mod580/cecdefull.htm. Accessed January 4, 2008.
6. Titler MG. Translation science: Quality, methods and issues. *Commun Nurs Res*. 2004;37:15,17–34.
7. Fraser I. Translation research: Where do we go from here? *Worldviews Evid Based Nurs*. 2004;1(S):S78–S83.
8. Oranta O, Routasalo P, Hupli M. Barriers to and facilitators of research utilization among Finnish registered nurses. *J Clin Nurs*. Mar 2002;11(2):205–213.
9. McCleary L, Brown GT. Barriers to paediatric nurses' research utilization. *J Adv Nurs*. May 2003;42(4):364–372.
10. Scott JG, Sochalski J, Aiken L. Review of magnet hospital research: Findings and implications for professional nursing practice. *J Nurs Adm*. 1999;29(1):9–19.
11. Larrabee JH, Janney M, Ostrow CL, et al. Predictors of registered nurse job satisfaction and intent to leave. *J Nurs Adm*. 2003;33(5):271–283.
12. Greenhalgh T, Robert G, Macfarlane F, et al. Diffusion of innovations in service organizations: Systematic review and recommendations. *Milbank Q*. 2004;82(4):581–629.
13. National League for Nursing. About the NLN. http://www.nln.org/aboutnln/index.htm. Accessed January 9, 2008.
14. American Nurses Association. About ANA. http:// www.nursingworld.org/FunctionalMenuCategories/AboutANA.aspx. Accessed January 9, 2008.

15. American Association of Critical-Care Nurses. Practice resources. http://www.aacn.org/AACN/practice.nsf/vwdoc/ StandardsforAcuteandCriticalCareNursingPractice. Accessed January 9, 2008.

16. American Nurses Association. Magnet Recognition Program. http://www.nursingworld.org/MainMenuCategories/Certification andAccreditation/Magnet.aspx. Accessed January 9, 2008.

17. Oncology Nursing Society. Evidence Based Practice Resource Area. http://onsopcontent.ons.org/toolkits/evidence/. Accessed January 9, 2008.

18. American Association of Critical-Care Nurses. Key statements, beliefs and philosophies behind the American Association of Critical-Care Nurses (AACN). http:// www.aacn.org/ AACN/memship.nsf/965028604675cdb88825680b006c88fa/ 7eda4030b16280f28825680a0071c4a8?OpenDocument. Accessed January 9, 2008.

19. National Council of State Boards of Nursing. Boards of Nursing. https://www.ncsbn.org/boards.htm. Accessed January 10, 2008.

20. American Association of Colleges of Nursing. About AACN. http://www.aacn.nche.edu/ContactUs/index.htm. Accessed January 10, 2008.

21. American Association of Colleges of Nursing. CCNE Accreditation. http://www.aacn.nche.edu/Accreditation/index.htm. Accessed January 10, 2008.

22. The Joint Commission. A Journey through the History of the Joint Commission. http://www.jointcommission.org/ AboutUs/ joint_commission_history.htm. Accessed January 10, 2008.

23. The Joint Commission. Certification of healthcare organizations. http://www.jointcommission.org/CertificationPrograms/. Accessed January 10, 2008.

24. Institute of Medicine. Institute of Medicine of the National Academies. http://www.iom.edu/. Accessed January 14, 2008.

25. Colton D. Quality improvement in health care. Conceptual and historical foundations. *Eval Health Prof.* Mar 2000;23(1):7–42.

26. Donabedian A. Evaluating the quality of medical care. *Milbank Mem Fund Q.* 1966;44(3, July, supplement):166–206.

27. Mitchell PH, Ferketich S, Jennings BM. Quality health outcomes model. American Academy of Nursing Expert Panel on Quality Health Care. *Image*. 1998;30(1):43–46.

28. Horsley J, Crane J, Crabtree MK, et al. *Using Research to Improve Nursing Practice: A Guide*. Orlando, FL: Grune & Stratton; 1983.

29. Stetler C, Marram G. Evaluating research findings for applicability in practice. *Nurs Outlook*. 1976;24(9):559–563.

30. Lindeman CA, Krueger JC. Increasing the quality, quantity, and use of nursing research. *Nurs Outlook*. Jul 1977;25(7):450–454.

31. Barnard KE, Hoehn RE. *Nursing Child Assessment Satellite Training: Final Report*. Hyattsville, MD: U.S. Department of Health, Education, and Welfare Division of Nursing; 1978.

32. Goode CJ, Lovett MK, Hayes JE, Butcher LA. Use of research based knowledge in clinical practice. *J Nurs Adm*. 1987;17(12):11–18.

33. Watson C, Bulechek G, McCloskey J. QAMUR: A quality assurance model using research. *J Nurs Care Qual*. 1987;2: 21–27.

34. Rosswurm MA. A research-based practice model in a hospital setting. *J Nurs Adm*. 1992;22(3):57–60.

35. Titler MG, Kleiber C, Steelman V, et al. Infusing research into practice to promote quality care. *Nurs Res*. 1994; 43(5): 307–313.

36. Dufault M. A collaborative model for research development and utilization: Process, structure, and outcomes. *J Nurs Staff Dev*. 1995;11(3):139–144.

37. Barnsteiner JH, Ford N, Howe C. Research utilization in a metropolitan children's hospital. *Nurs Clin North Am*. 1995;30(3):447–455.

38. Sackett DL, Rosenberg WM, Gray JA, et al. Evidence based medicine: What it is and what it isn't. *BMJ*. Jan 13 1996;312(7023):71–72.

39. Sackett DL. *Evidence-Based Medicine: How to Practice and Teach EBM*. 2nd ed. Edinburgh: Churchill Livingstone; 2000.

40. Rosswurm MA, Larrabee JH. A model for change to evidence-based practice. *Image J Nurs Sch*. 1999;31(4): 317–322.

41. Stetler CB. Updating the Stetler Model of Research Utilization to facilitate evidence-based practice. *Nurs Outlook.* 2001;49(6): 272–279.

42. Titler MG, Kleiber C, Steelman VJ, et al. The Iowa Model of Evidence-Based Practice to Promote Quality Care. *Crit Care Nurs Clin North Am.* 2001;13(4):497–509.

43. Soukup SM. The Center for Advanced Nursing Practice evidence-based practice model: Promoting the scholarship of practice. *Nurs Clin North Am.* Jun 2000;35(2):301–309.

44. Stevens KR. ACE Star Model of EBP: The Cycle of Knowledge Transformation. Academic Center for Evidence-based Practice. www.acestar.uthscsa.edu. Accessed August 21, 2003.

45. Rycroft-Malone J. The PARIHS framework—a framework for guiding the implementation of evidence-based practice. *J Nurs Care Qual.* Oct–Dec 2004;19(4):297–304.

46. Olade RA. Strategic collaborative model for evidence-based nursing practice. *Worldviews Evid Based Nurs.* 2004;1(1):60–68.

47. Newhouse R, Dearholt S, Poe S, et al. Evidence-based practice: A practical approach to implementation. *J Nurs Adm.* Jan 2005;35(1):35–40.

48. Rogers EM. *Diffusion of Innovations.* 4th ed. New York: Free Press; 1995.

49. Gustafson DH, Sainfort F, Eichler M, et al. Developing and testing a model to predict outcomes of organizational change. *Health Serv Res.* 2003;38(2):751–776.

50. Champagne F, Denis JL, Pineault R, Contandriopoulos AP. Structural and political models of analysis of the introduction of an innovation in organizations: The case of the change in the method of payment of physicians in long-term care hospitals. *Health Serv Manage Res.* Jul 1991;4(2):94–111.

51. Funk SG, Tornquist EM, Champagne MT. Barriers and facilitators of research utilization. An integrative review. *Nurs Clin North Am.* 1995;30(3):395–407.

52. Parahoo K. Barriers to, and facilitators of, research utilization among nurses in Northern Ireland. *J Adv Nurs.* Jan 2000; 31(1): 89–98.

53. Adams D. Breaking down the barriers: Perceptions of factors that influence the use of evidence in practice. *J Orthop Nurs.* 2001;5(4):170–175.

54. Titler MG, Cullen L, Ardery G. Evidence-based practice: An administrative perspective. *Reflect Nurs Leadersh.* 2002;28(2): 26–27, 46, 45.
55. Gifford W, Davies B, Edwards N, et al. Managerial leadership for nurses' use of research evidence: An integrative review of the literature. *Worldviews Evid Based Nurs.* 2007;4(3):126–145.
56. Stevens KR. *Essential Competencies for Evidence-Based Practice in Nursing.* San Antonio, TX: Academic Center for Evidence-Based Practice, University of Texas Health Science Center San Antonio; 2005.
57. Fanning MF, Oakes DW. A tool for quantifying organizational support for evidence-based practice change. *J Nurs Care Qual.* Apr–Jun 2006;21(2):110–113.
58. Larrabee JH, Sions J, Fanning M, et al. Evaluation of a program to increase evidence-based practice change. *J Nurs Adm.* 2007; 37(6):302–310.

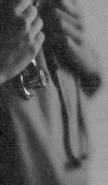

Chapter 2

THE MODEL FOR EVIDENCE-BASED PRACTICE CHANGE

OVERVIEW OF THE STEPS IN THE MODEL

The revised model is entitled the Model for Evidence-Based Practice Change, slightly different from the original model title of Model for Change to Evidence-Based Practice.[1] The new title was the one the authors of the original model had used when the manuscript was submitted for publication, but the name was changed in response to a reviewer recommendation. The reason for the renaming of the model was to emphasize *change,* using *evidence-based practice* to indicate the type of change. To the author, the title "Model for Change to Evidence-Based Practice" could imply a one-time change. The model has always been a model for planned *changes* in practice intended for use by nurses and other disciplines.

The revised schematic (Figure 2-1) was inspired by the author's experience with teaching and mentoring nurses in the

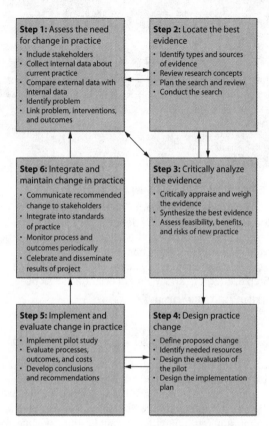

Step 1: Assess the need for change in practice
- Include stakeholders
- Collect internal data about current practice
- Compare external data with internal data
- Identify problem
- Link problem, interventions, and outcomes

Step 2: Locate the best evidence
- Identify types and sources of evidence
- Review research concepts
- Plan the search and review
- Conduct the search

Step 6: Integrate and maintain change in practice
- Communicate recommended change to stakeholders
- Integrate into standards of practice
- Monitor process and outcomes periodically
- Celebrate and disseminate results of project

Step 3: Critically analyze the evidence
- Critically appraise and weigh the evidence
- Synthesize the best evidence
- Assess feasibility, benefits, and risks of new practice

Step 5: Implement and evaluate change in practice
- Implement pilot study
- Evaluate processes, outcomes, and costs
- Develop conclusions and recommendations

Step 4: Design practice change
- Define proposed change
- Identify needed resources
- Design the evaluation of the pilot
- Design the implementation plan

Figure 2-1 Schematic for the Model for Evidence-Based Practice Change. Reprinted modified schematic from Rosswurm MA, Larrabee JH. A model for change to evidence-based practice. *Image J Nurs Sch.* 1999;31(4):317–322, with permission from Blackwell Publishing.

application of the original model since 1999, as well as prior experience with teaching and mentoring nurses in research utilization (RU).[2] The model remains a six-step model:

Step 1: Assess the need for change in practice.
Step 2: Locate the best evidence.
Step 3: Critically analyze the evidence.
Step 4: Design practice change.
Step 5: Implement and evaluate change in practice.
Step 6: Integrate and maintain change in practice.

The major changes from the original model are the combining of the original Steps 1 and 2 and the dividing of the original Step 3 into two steps: Step 2, locate the best evidence, and Step 3, critically analyze the evidence. Following is a brief description of the six steps.

Step 1: Assess the Need for Change in Practice

Major activities in this step are identifying and including the stakeholders of the practice problem; collecting internal data about the current practice; comparing the internal data with external data to confirm the need for a practice change; identifying the practice problem; and linking the problem, interventions, and outcomes. The teamwork tools used include structured brainstorming and multivoting on the practice problem. The use of applicable statistical process control tools is described. An example of a data collection instrument is included.

Step 2: Locate the Best Evidence

Major activities are identifying types and sources of evidence, reviewing research concepts, planning the search, and conducting the search. Included are tools for critically appraising qualitative and quantitative research studies, clinical practice guidelines, and systematic reviews. Also, examples of a table of evidence or a matrix for organizing the data about research studies prior to synthesis are included.

Step 3: Critically Analyze the Evidence

Major activities are critically appraising and weighing the strength of the evidence; synthesizing the best evidence; and assessing the feasibility, benefits, and risks of the new practice. Included are examples of completed critical appraisal forms for quantitative and qualitative research studies and systematic reviews. Also, examples of a completed table of evidence for quantitative and qualitative research studies are provided.

Step 4: Design Practice Change

Major activities include defining the proposed practice change, identifying the needed resources, designing the evaluation of the pilot, and designing the implementation plan. Change strategies described are the use of change champions, opinion leaders, educational sessions, educational materials, reminder systems, and audit and feedback.

Step 5: Implement and Evaluate Change in Practice

Major activities include implementing the pilot study; evaluating the processes, outcomes, and costs; and developing conclusions and recommendations.

Step 6: Integrate and Maintain Change in Practice

Major activities include communicating the recommended change to stakeholders, integrating the new practice into the standards of practice, monitoring the process and outcome indicators, and celebrating and disseminating the results of the project. Included are an example of a timeline template for preparing an annual calendar for multiple evidence-based practice (EBP) projects and an example of a completed calendar.

The revised schematic of the model illustrates that, although the steps are progressive, the model is not strictly linear. The two-way directional arrows between two steps indicate that the activities in each step may prompt activities in the other step.

For instance, suppose that an EBP team is searching for evidence on its project topic and finds very little evidence. The members would probably decide that they need to return to Step 1 and either refine their problem statement or clinical question or identify a different practice problem as the project focus. Suppose that in Step 3, as the team members are critically appraising the evidence, they decide that the evidence is weak. They may decide that they need to return to Step 2 and look for additional evidence or that they need to start over with Step 1. Suppose that in Step 5, as the team members are implementing the pilot study, they receive feedback from direct-care nurses that some aspect of the new practice is not working well. The team will troubleshoot and reconsider defining the new practice, a Step 4 activity. The arrow from Step 6 to Step 1 indicates that the ongoing monitoring of the process and outcomes indicators (Step 6) identifies the need for a new EBP project (Step 1) on a similar topic or a different topic.

TESTING OF THE MODEL

Nursing leaders at West Virginia University Hospitals (WVUH) initiated a systematic program of using research to improve patient-care quality in 1998 with the arrival of the Clinical Investigator, who functions in a joint-appointment role in both WVUH (25 percent) and the West Virginia University School of Nursing (WVUSON; 75 percent). A steering committee consisting of three directors and one manager worked with the Clinical Investigator in designing, implementing, and evaluating the research program. The two chief nurse executives (CNE) during the last eight years have been strong proponents of EBP, recognizing the many ways in which it adds value to the organization and ensuring the needed resources. The number of teams has fluctuated with the needs of the organization, ranging from five to nine. The teams conduct RU and EBP projects and are referred to as RU teams to distinguish them from the preexisting practice councils. Appendix 2-A is a cumulative list of topics for EBP projects conducted since 2000. Nine projects ended with the synthesis because there was not enough evidence to support a practice change. Nineteen projects led to practice changes, and eight projects are in progress. Several of the projects conducted the evaluation of the pilot as research studies.

The success of the WVUH nursing research program has been made possible by the CNE and the other nurse leaders creating mechanisms to support the various research-related activities. Budgeted time out of staffing has been critical to enable the work of the RU teams. A portion of the budget has covered the cost of subscriptions to several research journals and to full-text journals accessible from WVUH's intranet. Because of the affiliation with WVU, all nurses at WVUH also have access to WVU's electronic library resources. Furthermore, the budget included money to pay a "student worker" to retrieve article copies for RU teams and any WVUH nurse participating in research activities. This means that nurses have to actually go to the library only if they choose to do so. This student worker position was eliminated in 2007 because the WVU libraries' collection of full-text journals had increased sufficiently that teams were no longer giving requests for article retrieval to the student worker.

Nurses have had access to education and mentoring in conducting RU and EBP projects, as well as the research studies that have been conducted. The basic two-day workshop, taught by the Clinical Investigator, introduces participants to the nature of EBP, describes the Model for Change to Evidence-Based Practice,[1] gives them content and practice with critically appraising research, provides them with hands-on experience with searching the WVU electronic databases, and offers interactive exercises for applying the six steps of the model. This workshop is offered periodically when there are a sufficient number of nurses interested in attending.

A formal Nursing Research Council (NRC) was initiated in August 2003. The NRC is composed of one regular member and one alternate member from each of the six RU teams and representatives from nursing leadership (the CNE, four directors, two managers, the Clinical Investigator, and a second nurse researcher from the WVU School of Nursing). Team representatives give a report on their team's progress with their current topics. Members also discuss progress toward meeting the council's annual goals. A half-day retreat is held in late fall, during which council members discuss final progress on the annual goals and set new goals for the following year. The description of the nursing research program appears in Appendix 2-B.

Although the emphasis in our research program is on the use of best evidence to change practice, the program also supports and encourages the conduct of research. For instance, two direct-care nurses were the principal investigators on a pair of longitudinal quasi-experimental studies about the Children's Hospital's Baby-Friendly Hospital Initiative (BFHI): a one-year study on staff attitudes and practices, and a four-year study on mothers' attitudes and feeding practice and infant illness during the first year of life.

Information about the teams' projects and their products has been disseminated internally via the nursing division newsletter and posters. Furthermore, teams have disseminated information about their projects at peer-reviewed national and regional conferences and by publication in peer-reviewed professional journals. Our RU teams have begun receiving recognition for the high quality of their projects. For instance, during 2004, the Medical/Surgical RU Team received the Region 13 Sigma Theta Tau International Research Utilization Award for the bladder scanner project.

The RU teams' success has largely been due to interested nurses volunteering to serve and nurse leaders who cultivated nurses to be effective team members. As team members have become comfortable and skilled in conducting an RU or EBP project, they have also been instrumental in recruiting other members, mentoring each other, and keeping the team's momentum going.

The remaining six chapters of the book provide detailed descriptions of the six steps in the revised model. Cases are presented to illustrate key points.

REFERENCES

1. Rosswurm MA, Larrabee JH. A model for change to evidence-based practice. *Image J Nurs Sch*. 1999;31(4):317–322.
2. Larrabee JH. Achieving outcomes in a joint-appointment role. *Outcomes Manage*. 2001;5(2):52–56.
3. St. Clair K, Larrabee JH. Clean vs. sterile gloves: Which to use for postoperative dressing changes? *Outcomes Manage*. 2002;6(1):17–21.
4. Maramba PJ, Richards S, Myers AL, Larrabee JH. Discharge planning process: Applying a model for evidence-based practice. *J Nurs Care Qual*. Apr–Jun 2004;19(2):123–129.
5. Drenning C. Collaboration among nurses, advanced practice nurses, and nurse researchers to achieve evidence-based practice change. *J Nurs Care Qual*. Oct–Dec 2006;21(4):298–301.
6. Fanning MF. Reducing postoperative pulmonary complications in cardiac surgery patients with the use of the best evidence. *J Nurs Care Qual*. Apr–Jun 2004;19(2):95–99.
7. Anderson KL, Larrabee JH. Tobacco ban within a psychiatric hospital. *J Nurs Care Qual*. Jan–Mar 2006;21(1):24–29.
8. Sparks A, Boyer D, Gambrel A, et al. The clinical benefits of the bladder scanner: A research synthesis. *J Nurs Care Qual*. Jul–Sep 2004;19(3):188–192.
9. Richards T, Johnson J, Sparks A, Emerson H. The effect of music therapy on patients' perception and manifestation of pain, anxiety, and patient satisfaction. *Medsurg Nurs*. Feb 2007;16(1):7–14; quiz 15.
10. Horsley J, Crane J, Crabtree MK, et al. *Using Research to Improve Nursing Practice: A Guide*. Orlando, FL: Grune & Stratton; 1983.

Appendix 2-A   Research utilization and evidenced-based
practice change projects

West Virginia University Hospitals Nursing Division
2000–2007

Projects Ending With Synthesis
1. Clean vs. sterile gloves for postoperative wound
   dressing changes[3]
2. Family presence during crisis episode (Critical Care RU
   team)
3. Discharge planning by medical/surgical nurses
   (Medical/Surgical RU team)[4]
4. Cleanliness of perioperative environment (Perioperative
   RU team)
5. Preps with betadine paint vs. scrubs (Perioperative RU
   team)
6. Patient satisfaction regarding admission process
   (Oncology RU team)
7. Neutral field in the OR (Perioperative RU team)
8. Cord care (Children's Hospital RU team)
9. Advanced directives (Medical/Surgical RU team)[5]

Projects That Led To Practice Change
1. Baby-friendly hospital initiative to increase breastfeeding
   (Childrens Hospital RU team, research study completed,
   manuscript in progress)
2. Decreasing falls related to elimination needs
   (Medical/Surgical RU team)
3. Brushless surgical scrubs (Perioperative RU team)
4. Use of saline boluses before tracheal suctioning
   (Medical/Surgical RU team)
5. Incidence of postoperative pulmonary complications
   with using incentive spirometry in conjunction with early
   mobilization versus early mobilization alone (Critical
   Care RU team)[6]
6. Incidence of infection with shaving versus clipping in the
   preoperative cardiac surgery patient (Critical Care RU
   team)
7. Smoking and hospitalized psychiatric patients (Chestnut
   Ridge RU Team, research study)[7]

8. Sedation assessment of the intubated adult ICU patient (Critical Care RU team)
9. Patient satisfaction (Emergency Department RU team)
10. Chlorhexidine skin prep (Perioperative RU team)
11. Neonatal pain management (Children's Hospital RU team)
12. Child visitation (Critical Care RU team)
13. Oral care (Critical Care RU team)
14. Contraband and suicide precautions in psychiatry (Chestnut Ridge RU Team)
15. Use of bladder scanner to reduce urinary tract infections (Medical/Surgical RU team; research study)[8]
16. Impact of wrong site surgery protocol implementation (Perioperative RU team, research study completed, manuscript in progress)
17. Strategy to decrease contamination of enteral feedings (Critical Care RU team)
18. Groin dressing after percutaneous transluminal coronary angioplasty or stent sheath removal in critical care (Critical Care RU team, research study)
19. Fall risk assessment and falls prevention (Medical/Surgical RU team)

Projects in Progress
1. Feeding issues related to postoperative pediatric cardiac surgery (Childrens Hospital RU team)
2. Effectiveness of music therapy of reducing discomfort, pain, and anxiety (Medical/Surgical RU team)[9]
3. Pediatric and neonatal skin care and wound care (Childrens Hospital RU team)
4. Breast feeding and diabetes (research study)
5. Deep vein thrombophlebitis assessment and prevention (Medical/Surgical RU team; research study)
6. Preoperative management of glycemia in diabetic patients (Perioperative RU team)
7. Wisdom workers—registered nurse benefits and retention (Nursing Administration RU team)
8. Managing aggressive patients in psychiatry (Chestnut Ridge RU Team)

Appendix 2-B   West Virginia University Hospitals' Nursing
Research Program Description

West Virginia University Hospitals
Nursing Research Program

In keeping with the hospital's mission, philosophical beliefs, and management values, the Division of Nursing supports the conduct and utilization of clinically-oriented research and other best evidence.

Philosophical Beliefs Inherent in the Nursing Research Program
1. Research informs the pursuit of quality nursing care that can result in improved patient outcomes.
2. Staff participation in research activities fosters personal and professional development and enhances the quality of nursing practice.
3. Scientific integrity of research is enhanced by proposals meeting acceptability criteria.

Goals of the Nursing Research Program
The goals of the Nursing Research Program at WVU Hospitals are
1. To improve the quality of nursing care, patient outcomes, and patient perceptions of quality in a cost-effective manner
2. To foster best practice and
3. To enrich professional development.

Objectives of the Nursing Research Program
1. To utilize performance improvement (PI) findings in the identification of topics for RU or evidence-based practice (EBP) projects and research questions.
2. To conduct clinically relevant RU and EBP projects and research studies designed to inform nursing quality improvement.
3. To foster scientific problem-solving in practice, education, and management activities.
4. To support the acquisition of RU, EBP, and research conduct skills by Nursing Division staff.
5. To foster dissemination of findings from RU, EBP, and research projects by Nursing Division staff to local, state, and national audiences.

Nursing Research Program Activities
The Nursing Research Program at WVU Hospitals will include the conduct of RU and EBP projects to make best evidence practice changes, and, in selected cases, to conduct clinically relevant research studies.

A. Research Utilization and Evidence -BasedPractice
Research Utilization Teams will conduct RU and EBP projects of clinical relevance to the members' clinical site(s) on an on-going basis. Teams will consist of nursing staff and leaders, as well as representatives of other disciplines, as appropriate for the focus of a specific project. Teams will apply the Model for Change to Evidence Based Practice[1] in conducting the RU and EBP projects. This model includes "nonresearch" sources as evidence and acknowledges that, in some instances, such sources may be the best evidence available about the clinical focus of the project.

Research utilization is:
"A process directed toward the transfer of specific research-based knowledge into practice through the systematic use of a series of activities that include
1. identification and synthesis of multiple research studies that are related within a common conceptual base (research base);
2. transformation of the research-based knowledge into a clinical protocol that specifies nursing actions to meet specific patient care problems; and
3. implementation and evaluation of these nursing actions within nursing service organizations through the use of a planned change approach."[10, p. 100]

Evidence-based practice is the integration of:
"clinically relevant research, clinical expertise, and patient preference" when making decisions about effective, individualized patient care.[1, p. 317]

B. Research
The Nursing Division encourages the conduct of nursing research studies by its employees and external researchers. Both quantitative and qualitative research, as well as original and replication, research are encouraged.

1. Original research: An investigation, based on a conceptual framework, using formalized research strategies to describe, explain, predict, forecast, or control phenomena.
2. Replication research: An investigation that is a repetition of an original research, with or without modifications.

Organizational Structure of the Nursing Research Program

The Vice President for Nursing ensures that the Nursing Research Program reflects the hospital mission, philosophical beliefs, and management values. Figure 2-B.1 presents the organizational structure of the nursing research program. The Nursing Research Council reviews for approval all extramural research or research-related proposals, including those for students.

Members of the Nursing Research Council are responsible for the Nursing Research Program, with leadership and consultation from the Clinical Investigator who reports directly to the Vice President for Nursing. The Clinical Investigator serves as principle investigator for research studies of value to the organization and is responsible for dissemination of findings. The Clinical Investigator is responsible for mentoring Nursing Division staff in the utilization of research and other evidence in making practice changes designed to improve patient outcomes. The Clinical Investigator is also responsible for mentoring Nursing Division staff in the conduct of selected research studies, when appropriate.

The Nursing Research Council, whose members include staff nurses and nurse leaders, is responsible for oversight and guidance of the Division's RU and EBP initiatives. To that end, members will set annual goals and create mechanisms for achieving those goals. Also, in collaboration with the Clinical Investigator, the Council will design and implement formal and informal RU and EBP in-service activities. Council members are encouraged to initiate or participate collaboratively in research investigations and to consult with other staff regarding their utilization and conduct of research.

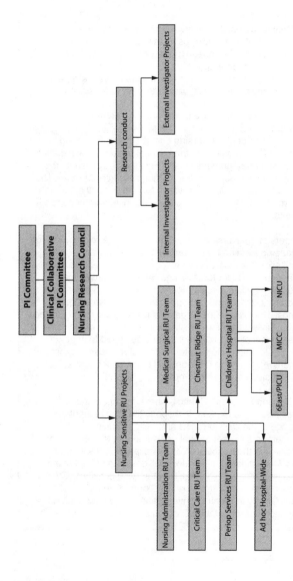

Figure 2-B.1   WVUH Clinical Collaborative Performance Improvement Chart

Functions of the Nursing Research Program

The nursing research program functions to achieve the program goals. The principal functions are:

1. To identify opportunities for improving practice using various sources of information, especially data from the Performance Improvement program.
2. To foster the acquisition and use of decision-making skills regarding RU and EBP by nursing division staff.
3. Conduct clinically-relevant research, when appropriate.
4. To modify standards of care based on research findings.
5. To improve practice through RU and EBP strategies and acquisition of new knowledge, including knowledge from translation science.

Policies of the Nursing Research Program

1. Any registered nurse employed by WVU Hospitals may submit a research proposal for approval.
2. All intramural proposals will be reviewed for approval by the Nursing Research Council.
3. The Director of the clinical service will review and approve any research proposal designed to include that service, regardless of the Principal Investigator's professional discipline.
4. All investigators must obtain University IRB approval of their research proposal prior to final approval by the Nursing Research Council and prior to initiation of the research.
5. Research consultation of students is the responsibility of their faculty.
6. Each investigator shall provide a follow-up report of their results to the Nursing Research Council and the Division of Nursing.

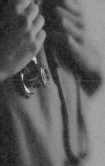

Chapter 3

STEP 1: ASSESS THE NEED FOR CHANGE IN PRACTICE

- **INCLUDE STAKEHOLDERS**
  - —Charter Team
  - —Determine Team Composition
  - —Assign Team Member Responsibilities
  - —Set Timelines
  - —Select Clinical Problem as Focus of Project
    - *Identify opportunities for improvement*
    - *Conduct brainstorming and multivoting*
      - *Consider parameters for prioritizing project topics*
      - *Confirm that an EBP project is the appropriate approach for solving the clinical problem*
      - *Conduct brainstorming*
        - *Unstructured brainstorming*
        - *Structured brainstorming*
      - *Conduct multivoting*

- **COLLECT INTERNAL DATA ABOUT CURRENT PRACTICE**
  - —Identify Data Sources
  - —Develop a Data Collection Instrument (DCI) and Collect Baseline Data
  - —Consider the Data Type Needed
  - —Decide on Sampling Plan and Sample Size
  - —Summarize Data and Interpret Results

- **COMPARE EXTERNAL DATA WITH INTERNAL DATA**
  - —Conduct Informal Benchmarking
  - —Consider Available Formal Benchmarking Programs
  - —Benchmark against Published Literature
- **IDENTIFY THE PROBLEM**
- **LINK PROBLEM, INTERVENTIONS, AND OUTCOMES**
  - —Use Standardized Classification Systems and Language
  - —Identify Potential Interventions
  - —Select Outcome Indicators
  - —Develop a Specific Goal for the evidence-based practice (EBP) Project
  - —Setting EBP Project Goal without Using Standardized Languages
    - *Informal use of the nursing process*
    - *Asking answerable questions*

INCLUDE STAKEHOLDERS

Charter Team

An ad hoc EBP team may be chartered to conduct one project. In some cases, an EBP project may be conducted by one nurse with unique expertise or interest, with input from the rest of the EBP team. More commonly, an EBP team is chartered to conduct a series of projects for its designated clinical area, with the membership composition being adjusted based on the clinical focus of the project.

 CASE 3-1 *Clean vs. Sterile Gloves*

The first EBP project[1] conducted at West Virginia University Hospitals (WVUH) was assigned to one staff nurse, who was awarded a nursing research fellowship with six weeks paid time out of staffing to conduct the project. The Clinical Investigator mentored her in the process and skills needed to conduct the project. She explored the evidence to determine the safety of using clean rather than sterile gloves in postoperative wound dressing changes. This topic warranted examination because two surgeons had been advising nurses to abandon the hospital policy of using only sterile gloves during postoperative wound dressing changes. Some of the nurses were uncomfortable with abandoning the current standard of care. Once the nurse had completed a review of current practice and a summary of the literature, she met with a small hospitalwide ad hoc team to present and discuss her recommendations. Those recommendations included re-educating the staff on the need to follow the existing policy of using sterile gloves because the evidence did not support a change to using clean gloves. The ad hoc team's responsibilities for the project were limited to discussing and approving the recommendations. In all subsequent projects, team members had more substantive responsibilities, even when a team member was awarded a nursing research fellowship to do a portion of the project.

Determine Team Composition

Team composition is a critical consideration. Project success, in part, is dependent upon there being representation of all stakeholders of the practice. Potential stakeholders include nurses, nurse leaders, physicians, other health-care disciplines, patients, and the patients' family members. In a project aimed at reducing postoperative pulmonary complications in cardiac surgery patients, the team members included nurses, nurse managers, the nursing director, physicians, and respiratory therapists.[2] As the team deliberates about the topic for the project, members appropriate for the topic chosen are added. Although it may not be feasible to include patients or their family members as EBP team members, the team can obtain the ideas or concerns that patients or their family members have about their care through informal surveys or by inviting them to participate in a focus group.

Assign Team Member Responsibilities

The team leader may be elected by the membership or appointed by a nurse administrator. The team leader is responsible for preparing and distributing the meeting agenda prior to the meetings. The group also must decide who will be responsible for minute taking. This may be a rotating responsibility among members, or there may be one designated member or clerical staff person. Expectations about the timeliness of minutes preparation must be determined. Because of these structural decisions, the team's first meeting may be organizational. If the team is given a charter to focus on a specific clinical topic for its project, its members discuss this charter for clarification. If the charter is to improve outcomes for an important aspect of care that they identify, the team defines the charter by the end of Step 1. Also by the end of Step 1, team members should decide on the division of labor among themselves. Some may volunteer to conduct the search for evidence, while others will retrieve the references, critique the references, or write a synthesis from the evidence. Others will take the lead in designing and conducting the pilot for the new practice.

Set Timelines

Once it is decided that an EBP project will be conducted, the team assembles to plan the project timeline and to deliberate on the topic for the EBP project. Conducting an EBP project is resource intensive and takes time. Depending on the nature of the project and the source of the evidence, most EBP projects will take 6 to 12 months to conduct. Figure 3-1 displays a sample timeline or Gantt chart. While timelines are intended to provide structure for the team's work, they should also be considered flexible. It is not always possible to foresee circumstances that will delay activities within a step of the model. Team members who are health-care providers retain health-care delivery responsibilities while participating in the project. Other team members also have competing demands on their time. At the end of each step in the model, team members should evaluate their progress and adjust the timeline for the remaining steps in the model if necessary.

Tasks	Duration*	Start	Finish	Completed
Step 1: Assess need for change in practice (define topic)	35 days			
-Collect internal data about current practice	25 days			
-Compare external with internal data	5 days			
-Identify problem	5 days			
-Link problem, interventions, and outcomes	1 day			
Step 2: Locate the best evidence	50 days			
Plan the search	5 days			
Conduct the search	45 days			
Step 3: Critically analyze the evidence	75 days			
-Critically appraise and weigh the evidence	20 days			
-Synthesize best evidence	20 days			
-Assess feasibility, benefits, and risks of new practice	5 days			
Step 4: Design practice change	60 days			
-Design proposed change	5 days			
-Identify needed resources	5 days			
-Design the evaluation of the pilot	5 days			
-Design the implementation plan	10 days			
Step 5: Implement & evaluate practice change	80 days			
-Implement pilot study	60 days			
-Evaluate processes, outcomes, and costs	20 days			
-Develop conclusions and recommendations	5 days			
Step 6: Integrate & maintain change in practice	50 days			
-Communicate recommended change to stakeholders	10 days			
-Integrate into standards of practice	30 days			
-Monitor process and outcomes periodically	10 days			
-Celebrate and disseminate results of project	90 days			

*These are estimates and vary with the nature of the project.

Figure 3-1   Timeline template 1.

lect Clinical Problem as Focus of Project

dentify opportunities for improvement

Having chartered a team, assembled members, set timelines, and completed the organizing meeting, the EBP team launches the discussion about the clinical focus of the project. Initiation of an EBP project may be prompted by a variety of factors, including

- A nurse's judgment, based on critical reflection, that there is an opportunity for improvement in a practice and its outcomes
- A new "hot topic" or new standard from the Joint Commission or another accrediting agency
- A new standard of practice released by a professional organization such as the American Nurses Association or the American Association of Critical-Care Nurses
- Publication of a new clinical practice guideline, systematic review, or research report that nurses judge to be important to their clinical practice
- A quarterly report of adverse events
- The occurrence of a "sentinel event," meaning an adverse event with such dire consequences that each one must be scrutinized for causes
- A complaint about care from patients, families, physicians, or other health-care providers

Conduct brainstorming and multivoting

Consider parameters for prioritizing project topics

While making a choice about the clinical focus of the project, the following should be considered. Is the clinical focus or practice

- High risk, problem-prone, or high volume?
- Using more resources than the anticipated reimbursement?
- High priority to the organization's mission, vision, and values?

Confirm that an EBP project is the appropriate approach for solving the clinical problem

Because an EBP project is resource intensive, team members must justify the topic selection by asking themselves if an EBP change is the best approach to take for solving the clinical problem. It is not, if

- The problem requires an immediate solution; that would require a rapid management approach.
- The problem is failure to follow existing standards; that requires a management solution aimed at increasing staff adherence to existing standards.
- The solution does not require scientific evidence; that problem may require a continuous quality improvement approach.

An EBP project is appropriate if the topic involves a clinical problem for which scientific evidence exists. Keeping these parameters in mind, the team moves into the process of selecting the clinical focus for the EBP project.

Conduct brainstorming

Unstructured brainstorming

- Purpose: idea generation for the clinical focus of the project
- Process:
    — Display the central brainstorming question
        - Example: "What patient outcome or aspect of care in our unit (division, hospital) most needs improvement?"
- Discuss ideas, without guidelines for the process

Structured brainstorming [3]

- Purpose: idea generation, maximizing creativity and minimizing criticism and domination by the most vocal
- Process:
    — Decide on the central brainstorming question and display it for all to see.
        - Example: "What patient outcome or aspect of care in our unit (division, hospital) most needs improvement?"

○ Nighttime falls by elderly patients due to "sundowner's" syndrome and toileting needs
○ Inadequate continuity of care due to more than three lateral transfers during hospitalization
○ Unplanned readmission of chronic heart failure patients less than 30 days after discharge due to inadequate self-care
○ Phlebitis due to nurse noncompliance with peripheral IV therapy policy
○ Late medication administration due to chronic pharmacy delivery delays
○ Inadequate diabetes management on day of surgery due to lack of a protocol
○ Patient dissatisfaction with pain management

Figure 3-2   Sample list of clinical topics generated during structured brainstorming in response to the brainstorming question "What patient outcome or aspect of care in our unit most needs improvement?"

- Members spend five to ten minutes silently writing down all of their own thoughts about the question.
  — Sequentially, in turn, each member shares one idea. No idea is criticized. The only discussion is for clarification, and that is led by the team leader.
  — The cycle of sharing one idea at a time continues until each person passes, having exhausted his or her list of ideas.
  — Team leader:
    ▪ Writes each idea on a flip chart using the exact words of the contributor (Figure 3-2)
    ▪ Clarifies each idea
    ▪ Helps the team discard duplicate ideas and confirm that the problem warrants an EBP approach
    ▪ Writes out the final list on a new sheet of flip chart paper, assigning an alphabetic letter as a label (Figure 3-3)

Conduct multivoting
- Purpose: to achieve team consensus on the prioritization of clinical topics for which improvement opportunities exist.

A Nighttime falls by elderly patients due to "sundowner's" syndrome and toileting needs

B Inadequate continuity of care due to more than three lateral transfers during hospitalization

C Unplanned readmission of chronic heart failure patients less than 30 days after discharge due to inadequate self-care

X Phlebitis due to nurse noncompliance with peripheral IV therapy policy—*refer for a management solution*

X Late medication administration due to chronic pharmacy delivery delays—*refer for a continuous quality improvement solution*

D Inadequate diabetes management on day of surgery due to lack of a protocol

E Patient dissatisfaction with pain management

Figure 3-3   Clinical topic list for multivoting.

Gives each team member equal opportunity to participate in topic selection for the EBP project.

- Process:
  — Each member
    ▪ Records the corresponding letters for each topic on a piece of paper.
    ▪ Assigns a rank order to each topic, with the highest number being most important.
      ○ For example, if the list has five responses, the most important will be ranked as 5, the next most important as 4, and so on.
  — Team leader
    ▪ Sums the rankings from all team members on the flip chart page (Figure 3-4).
- The topic with the highest group ranking is C: Unplanned readmission of chronic heart failure (CHF) patients less than 30 days after discharge due to inadequate self-care.
- The team would work on this clinical practice problem first, collecting internal data about the current practice and comparing those data with external data to verify the need for improvement.

Topic	Jane	Mike	Bill	SUM
A	5	3	2	10
B	4	4	1	9
C	3	5	5	13
D	2	2	4	8
E	1	1	3	5

Figure 3-4　Ballot for multivoting.

COLLECT INTERNAL DATA ABOUT CURRENT PRACTICE

Identify Data Sources

Team members collect internal data about the current practice that are pertinent to the clinical problem. These data may come from existing data sources, including

- Risk management databases
- Infection control databases
- Clinical information systems
- Patient satisfaction surveys
- Staff or physician surveys
- Agency-specific reports of performance on quality indicators
- Financial databases

 CASE 3-2　*Chronic Heart Failure*

For the topic selected through multivoting, unplanned readmission of CHF patients less than 30 days after discharge due to inadequate self-care, the team would need to obtain data about the volume of CHF patients who were readmitted less than 30 days after discharge during the previous 12 months.

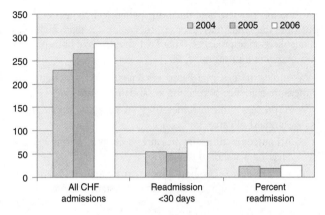

Figure 3-5   Histogram displaying unplanned readmissions of CHF patients <30 days after discharge (data fabricated).

Those data should be available from personnel working with existing clinical data sets. In the fabricated CHF example, the team obtained data on all CHF admissions and unplanned CHF admissions less than 30 days after discharge for three consecutive years. Based on these data, the team determined that the volume of CHF patients who were readmitted in less than 30 days was higher than desired (Figure 3-5).

Develop a Data Collection Instrument (DCI) and Collect Baseline Data

When there are no existing data sources pertaining to the clinical problem, the team should develop a DCI and collect baseline data. For instance, obtaining baseline data for Case 3-2 about CHF patients' knowledge about self-care after discharge and relevant teaching by registered nurses (RNs) would require the development of a DCI and data collection. If the information needed is about staff practice only, the DCI could be a simple questionnaire with open- and closed-ended questions. If the information needed is about both patient outcomes and staff practice, the team may choose observation or chart review as data collection approaches. That DCI should have both process and outcome indicators.

- An indicator is a rate-based statement that is designed to measure evidence of meeting a standard of care.
  - A process indicator measures an action specified by a standard of care.
  - An outcome indicator measures a desired consequence of meeting a standard of care.
    - All EBP projects should focus on a patient outcome, but may also include cost of care or system outcomes.

 CASE 3-2.A *Chronic Heart Failure*

A sample of a DCI for collecting chart review data about CHF nursing care is displayed in Figure 3-6. This form is designed to collect data on one patient. Process and outcome indicators are clearly identified.

A sample of a DCI for collecting observation and chart review data about a Foley care standard of practice is displayed in Figure 3-7. This form is designed to collect data on up to 10 patients with a Foley catheter on one unit. The three observation indicators and the first chart review indicator are process indicators. The second chart review indicator, as stated, is an outcome indicator.

Consider the Data Type Needed

When designing a DCI, the team needs to consider the type of data needed. When possible, it should develop indicators that produce continuous data rather than discrete data.

- Discrete data are qualitative values that occur in a finite or limited range. Discrete data are produced by
  - Nominal scales, which assign a number to represent characteristics of people or things.

Chart Review Form: Chronic Heart Failure Nursing Care		
ID#: _____		

ANSWER CODE:

1 = YES	0 = NO	ND = Not Documented	NA = Not Applicable

SOURCE CODE:

A. Flowsheet	D. CHF Order Set	G. Staff Notes
B. CANOPY*	E. Patient Registration Form	H. Discharge Summary
C. Plan of care form	F. Blue Sheet	

			SOURCE
	Date chart reviewed?		Write in
	Amount of time needed to complete this chart review?		Write in
	Medical Record/Account Number		E
	Discharge Date		F
	Year first diagnosed with CHF		Hx & PE
	CRITERIA	**ANSWER**	
	Process Indicators		
1.	Did the physician use the CHF Order Set?		B, D
2.	RN performed initial assessment within 8 hours of admission?		C
3.	a) How many times *should* nurse have performed every 8-hour assessment?		F
	b) How many times did nurse *actually* perform every 8-hour assessment?		A
	% compliance		3B/3A
4.	Did the patient demonstrate any key changes in health status?		A, B
	If NO, skip to question 5		
	If YES		
	a) How many times did key changes in health status occur?		A
	b) For how many of those times did the RN notify the physician so that the plan of care could be changed?		A
	% compliance		4B/4A

Figure 3-6   Sample of data collection instrument for a chart review pertaining to CHF nursing care.

5.	Did the RN document patient need for Social Services for discharge planning?		B, C
	If NO, skip to question 6		
	a) If **YES**, was a Social Services consult ordered?		D
	% compliance		5A/5
6.	Did the RN document patient need for Physical Therapy?		B, C
	If NO, skip to question 7		
	a) If **YES**, was a Physical Therapy consult ordered?		D
	% compliance		6A/6
7.	RN taught patient self-care needed after discharge for		
	a) medicines		A, D, H
	b) weight management (fluid restrictions)		A, D, H
	c) signs and symptoms needing physician attention		A, D, H
	Discharge Outcome Indicators		
8.	Lung sounds improved since admission?		A, B
9.	O^2 saturation 88% or higher while on:		
	a) Room air		A, B
	b) O^2		A, B
10.	Patient states he/she knows to report to physician		
	a) 2.5 pound (or individualized amount) weight gain		H, D
	b) SOB with usual activity		H, D
	c) other individualized discharge instructions		H, D

*Case management notes

Figure 3-6   (*Continued*)

- Example 1: Indicator 1 in Figure 3-7, "Foley catheter attached to leg strap"
  - Response choices are only 1 (yes) or 0 (no).
  - Data for which there are only two possible values are also referred to as binomial.
- Example 2:
  - Smoking history
    - 0 = Never smoked

Unit _____
Date _____

Observation Data							Answer Code: 1 = Yes			0 = No	
Patient	1	2	3	4	5	6	7	8	9	10	SUM
1. Foley catheter attached to leg strap											
2. Foley insertion site clean											
3. Foley catheter positioned correctly to prevent reflux											

Documentation Data							Answer Code: 1 = Yes			0 = No	
Patient	1	2	3	4	5	6	7	8	9	10	SUM
1. Foley care documented every shift											
2. Foley catheter dwell time is less than 30 days											

Figure 3-7 Sample data collection instrument for Foley catheter care.

- 1 = Has quit now but smoked at least 1 pack of cigarettes per week for at least 1 year
- 2 = Still smoking and smoked at least 1 pack of cigarettes per week for at least 1 year
  - Note that the assigned numbers for the responses have qualitative, not quantitative, value.

— Ordinal scales, which assign a number to represent categories of a characteristic that are arranged in a meaningful order, such as from low to high. Likert-type scales produce ordinal data.

- Example: Select the number that best indicates the severity of your pain right now:
  - 0 = no pain
  - 1 = very little pain
  - 2 = mild pain
  - 3 = moderate pain
  - 4 = severe pain
- Note that the numbers represent sequential changes in pain intensity, but the difference in quantitative value between one number and the next is unknown.

• Continuous data are quantitative values that occur in an infinite or unlimited range. Continuous data are produced by

— Interval scales, which assign a number to represent ordered categories of a characteristic for which the intervals between the numbers are equal; however, the zero point is arbitrary, and therefore an interval scale cannot provide information about the exact magnitude of the differences between points on the scale.

- Example: Temperature measurement involves scales with arbitrary zero points.

— Ratio scales, which assign a number to represent meaningfully ordered categories of a characteristic for which the intervals between the numbers are equal and the scale has a true zero.

- Example 1: measurement of
  - weight
  - pulse
  - blood pressure
- Example 2: Indicator 3 in Figure 3-6
  - 3a. How many times *should* the nurse have performed every 8-hour assessment? This is a denominator.
  - 3b. How many times did the nurse *actually* perform every 8-hour assessment? This is a numerator.
  - Percent compliance is obtained by dividing the response to 3b. by the response to 3a.
    - Note that this approach to measurement produces more precise data than an indicator that asks whether or not the nurse performed the every 8-hour assessment.

Decide on Sampling Plan and Sample Size

Obtaining data from the entire population is a costly and time-consuming task. When conducting quality improvement monitoring and EBP projects, the EBP team may need to obtain data from the entire population of interest if that population consists of patients who have experienced a sentinel event or other adverse occurrence. For other topics, it is usually impractical to obtain data for the entire population of interest. Rather, the EBP team's goal should be to obtain data that are representative of the population of interest. The team decides on the population of interest while selecting the topic for the EBP project. In the multivoting example discussed in this chapter (Case 3-2), the selected topic was "unplanned readmission of CHF patients less than 30 days after discharge due to inadequate self-care." Thus, the population of interest is patients admitted with CHF, a high-volume diagnosis in acute-care and regional access hospitals. The team must decide on the sampling plan to use when collecting data.

The sampling plan with the least chance of being representative of the population is convenience sampling, meaning that the team collects data from all available CHF patients who agree to participate within a specified time frame. Random selection is much more likely to produce a representative sample. Coin tossing and drawing numbers out of a hat are quick, simple approaches to random selection when the population of interest is not large. If the team wanted to sample closed charts of CHF patients hospitalized in the last 12 months, the use of a table of random numbers would be a more practical approach to random selection.

The team must also decide on the sample size. The Joint Commission[4] requires the following sample sizes when collecting data about structure or process elements of a standard of care, and these guidelines may be used when deciding on sample size for the EBP project evaluation:

- "for a population of
  — fewer than 30 cases, sample 100% of available cases
  — 30 to 100 cases, sample 30 cases
  — 101 to 500 cases, sample 50 cases
  — greater than 500 cases, sample 70 cases"

For greater confidence that the size will be adequate, the team should consider using sample size calculator software. There are a number of web sites with access to statistical software. One web site that includes sample size calculators is http://statpages.org/

There are introductory statistics books available should members of an EBP team wish to begin developing an understanding of statistics, including sample size calculation.[5,6] Some health-care organizations may have a decision support department that can perform the sample size calculation. If the team plans to conduct the evaluation component of the project as a research study, the members should consult with someone who has statistical expertise about appropriate sample size. If there is no resource person in the organization who can perform the power analysis, the EBP team should explore the possibility of finding a statistician to serve as a consultant. One approach would be to browse the web site of the Department of Statistics or the Department of Mathematics at a local or regional university.

Summarize Data and Interpret Results

Once data collection is completed, the EBP team members need to summarize the data and display the results preliminary to discussing and interpreting the data. The data may be entered into data management software such as Excel. The team should use the services of the decision support department or other organization resources with skill in data management, if available.

 CASE 3-2.b *Chronic Heart Failure*

Figure 3-8 displays an Excel file with fabricated data for indicators pertaining to RN teaching for 30 CHF patients. Responses to the indicators were either yes or no (discrete, binomial data). Formulas inserted into the COUNT, SUM, and PERCENT rows performed the calculations. The formula for percent included dividing the SUM by the COUNT and multiplying by 100. This made it possible to convert discrete data from individuals to continuous data for the sample. For this fabricated sample of 30 CHF patients, the RN had taught 73.3 percent of patients about own medicines, 10 percent about weight management, and 23.3 percent about signs and symptoms to report to the physician. Results for the outcomes indicators were that 16.7 percent of the sample knew to report a weight gain of 2.5 pounds and 30 percent knew to report shortness of breath. There were no quantitative results for the indicator pertaining to the patient knowing other individualized discharge instructions because there was no documentation, suggesting that this knowledge was not assessed.

Patient	Taught meds	Taught wt management	Taught S&S	Knows wt management	Knows SOB	Knows other
1	1	0	0	0	0	ND
2	1	0	0	0	0	ND
3	0	0	0	0	0	ND
4	1	0	0	0	1	ND
5	1	1	1	0	0	ND
6	1	0	1	0	0	ND
7	1	0	1	1	1	ND
8	1	0	0	0	0	ND
9	0	0	0	0	0	ND
10	1	0	0	0	0	ND
11	1	0	0	0	0	ND
12	1	0	0	0	0	ND
13	1	0	0	0	0	ND
14	1	0	0	0	0	ND
15	1	0	0	0	1	ND
16	1	0	1	1	1	ND
17	1	0	1	0	1	ND
18	0	0	0	0	1	ND
19	1	0	0	0	0	ND
20	0	0	0	0	0	ND
21	0	1	1	1	1	ND
22	1	0	0	0	0	ND
23	0	0	0	0	0	ND
24	1	0	0	1	1	ND
25	1	0	0	1	0	ND
26	0	0	0	0	0	ND
27	1	0	0	0	0	ND
28	1	0	0	0	1	ND
29	1	1	0	0	0	ND
30	0	0	1	0	0	ND
COUNT	30	30	30	30	30	0
SUM	22	3	7	5	9	
PERCENT	73.3	10.0	23.3	16.7	30.0	

Figure 3-8   Excel spreadsheet displaying indicator data for chronic heart failure nursing care study ($n = 30$) for patients hospitalized during the fourth quarter of 2006 (data fabricated).

CASE 3-2.C *Chronic Heart Failure*

Figure 3-9 displays fabricated results for all process and outcome indicators on the DCI for CHF nursing care by simply using a copy of the DCI on which one column was relabeled "Frequency (%)" and a second column was relabeled "Mean (SD, standard deviation)." By examining these results, the EBP team can confirm that there is an opportunity for improving several aspects of nursing care for CHF patients, including teaching patients the information they need for self-care after discharge.

The team may wish to know how the results from this data set compare with data from the previous year or two. By collecting data from charts of CHF patients hospitalized in the fourth quarter of the previous two years and entering them into Excel, the team can generate charts that visually display the results for the three time points. Using a run chart, Figure 3-10 displays the results at three time points for the indicators pertaining to teaching the CHF patient and the patients' knowledge about information needed for self-care after discharge. Figure 3-11 displays the same information in a histogram chart. Both make it easy to see several things:

- RNs performed best on teaching CHF patients about their medicines.
- Performance on teaching patients about their medicines has improved since 2004; however
  — That performance decreased between 2005 and 2006
  — It has not approached 100 percent
- Performance on teaching patients about weight management and when to report signs and symptoms to the physician warrant marked improvement.
- Patients were more knowledgeable about reporting shortness of breath to the physician than about reporting weight gain, however:
  — Slightly less than one-third knew to report shortness of breath
  — That knowledge appears unrelated to RNs' teaching about signs and symptoms to report.

		Frequency (%)	Mean (SD)
	Amount of time needed to complete this chart review?		32 (7) minutes
	CRITERIA		
	Process Indicators		
1.	Did the physician use the CHF Order Set?	18 (60%)	
2.	RN performed initial assessment within 8 hours of admission?	30 (100%)	
3.	a) How many times *should* nurse have perform every 8-hour assessment?	96	
	b) How many times nurse *actually* performed every 8-hour assessment?	72	
	% compliance	75%	
4.	Did the patient demonstrate any key changes in health status?	5 (16.7%)	
	If NO, skip to question 5		
	If YES		
	a) How many times did key changes in health status occur?	5	
	b) For how many of those times did the RN notify the physician so that the plan of care could be changed?	5 (100%)	
5.	Did the RN document patient need for Social Services for discharge planning?	8	
	If NO, skip to question 6		
	a) If **YES,** was a Social Services consult ordered?	8 (100%)	
6.	Did the RN document patient need for Physical Therapy?	3	
	If NO, skip to question 7		
	a) If **YES,** was a Physical Therapy consult ordered?	3 (100%)	
7.	RN taught patient self-care needed after discharge for		
	a) medicines	22 (73.3%)	
	b) weight management (fluid restrictions)	3 (10%)	
	c) signs and symptoms needing physician attention	7 (23.3%)	
	Discharge Outcome Indicators		
8.	Lung sounds improved since admission?	30 (100%)	
9.	O^2 saturation 88% or higher while on:		
	a) Room air	24 (80%)	
	b) O^2	6 (20%)	
10.	Patient states he/she knows to report to physician		
	a) 2.5 pound (or individualized amount) weight gain	5 (16.7%)	
	b) SOB with usual activity	9 (30%)	
	c) other individualized discharge instructions	NA – none documented	

Figure 3-9   Summary for chronic heart failure nursing care study ($n = 30$) for patients hospitalized during the fourth quarter of 2006 (data fabricated).

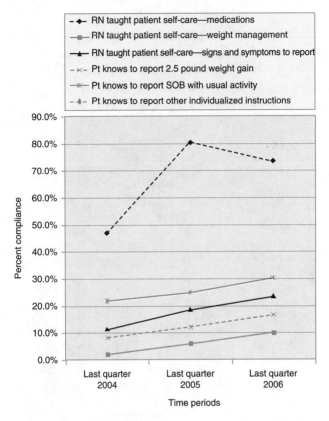

Figure 3-10 Run chart displaying percent compliance with the standard of nursing care for chronic heart failure and relevant patient knowledge outcomes (data fabricated). SOB, shortness of breath.

This example demonstrates internal benchmarking, the comparison of internal data at two or more time points. More detailed information on the purpose and use of statistical process control (SPC) tools, such as run charts and Pareto

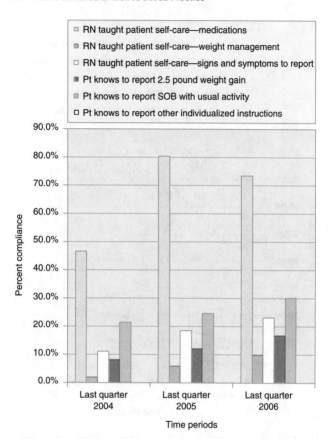

Figure 3-11   Histogram displaying percent compliance with the standard of nursing care for chronic heart failure and relevant patient knowledge outcomes (data fabricated). SOB, shortness of breath.

charts, and teamwork tools is available in the literature.[3,7,8] Internal benchmarking enables the team to examine the data for trends over time. Once the team has performed internal benchmarking, the next activity is external benchmarking.

COMPARE INTERNAL DATA WITH EXTERNAL DATA

Conduct Informal Benchmarking

Benchmarking, or comparing internal data with external data, enables the team to verify opportunities for improvement and to set goals. Benchmarking may be done informally or through formal benchmarking programs. Informal benchmarking may consist of collecting data from similar health-care agencies regarding their outcomes and relevant practice. When using an informal process, the team members should develop an interview guide with specific questions so that they obtain responses to those questions from each comparison agency.

Consider Available Formal Benchmarking Programs

The number of formal benchmarking programs available has increased over the past two decades. Examples include:

- The Joint Commission–ORYX Core Performance Measures[9]: participating hospitals receive periodic benchmarked reports on their performance on standards of care.
- Centers for Medicare and Medicaid Services—Quality Initiatives:[10]
  — Home care quality initiatives: these include monitoring of indicators using the Outcome and Assessment Information Set (OASIS)
    ■ Home health compare[11]: searchable benchmarked reports about performance on the following quality indicators for home health-care agencies:
      ○ Improvement in ambulation/locomotion
      ○ Improvement in bathing
      ○ Improvement in transferring
      ○ Improvement in management of oral medication

- Improvement in pain interfering with activity
- Acute-care hospitalization
- Emergent care
- Discharge to community
- Improvement in dyspnea (shortness of breath)
- Improvement in urinary incontinence

— Hospital quality initiatives

  - Hospital compare: searchable benchmarked reports about performance on the following quality indicators for hospitals[12]:
    - Acute myocardial infarction
    - Heart failure
    - Pneumonia
    - Surgical care improvement/surgical infection prevention
  - Premier hospital initiative demonstration: participating hospitals receive bonus Medicare payments for high performance on the following quality indicators. Benchmarked reports are available online.
    - Acute myocardial infarction
    - Heart failure
    - Community-acquired pneumonia
    - Coronary artery bypass graft
    - Knee and hip replacement

• American Nurses Association, National Center for Nursing Quality[13]

  — National Database of Nursing Quality Indicators, a proprietary database with nurse-sensitive quality indicators, including

    - Patient falls
    - Pain management
    - Pressure ulcers
    - Peripheral IV infiltration

— Unit-specific reports, showing comparisons to similar units, are given to participating hospitals every quarter.

- University HealthSystem Consortium[14]
    — An alliance of academic medical centers and their affiliated hospitals that can choose to participate in clinical benchmarking projects

Benchmark against Published Literature

Often, there are no external databases available for external benchmarking of nurse-sensitive clinical problems. In such cases, the team must rely on published literature or informal benchmarking, or a combination of the two. For the CHF example (Case 3-2), there is evidence in the research literature of higher scores on comparable teaching performance indicators and patient knowledge of self-care, providing further justification for focusing on the clinical problem of unplanned readmission of CHF patients less than 30 days after discharge due to inadequate self-care. After completing external benchmarking, the team drafts a statement of the practice problem.

IDENTIFY THE PROBLEM

During the structured brainstorming example discussed earlier in this chapter, seven potential topics were identified for the clinical practice problem. Before multivoting occurred, clarification led by the team leader identified one topic as needing a management approach and another topic as needing a continuous quality improvement approach, leaving five potential topics from which to choose one that would be the focus of the EBP project. Having completed internal and external benchmarking, the team now discusses whether or not the initial statement of the clinical problem is sufficiently descriptive. In the CHF example, the internal data confirmed that there were opportunities for reducing the number of unplanned readmissions, increasing RN teaching of information needed by CHF

Step 1. Assess need for change in practice
- The MSRUT identified the stakeholders as patients, nurses, physicians, nursing leaders, and Materials Management personnel.
- Current nursing practice for urinary retention and postvoid residual checks was urinary catheterization.
- The problem identified was frequent urinary tract infections (UTIs) in the acute-care population. UTI rates in all participating units showed an opportunity for improvement.
- The MSRUT consulted with nurses from another health-care organization who had implemented a bladder-scanning program.

Step 2. Link problem with interventions and outcomes
- The MSRUT linked the problem with an intervention and selected desired outcomes.
- The selected intervention was to use the bladder scanner before a urinary catheterization procedure.
- The clinical outcome indicator selected for evaluation was a decrease in the number of UTIs.

Step 3. Synthesize best evidence
- The MSRUT completed a synthesis of the best evidence. An extensive literature search related to the use of bladder scanners was completed.[39]
- The MSRUT assessed the feasibility, benefits, and risks of using bladder scanners in the acute-care setting.
- The benefits included: possible decrease in the number of urinary catheterizations and UTIs, patient comfort, less embarrassment for patients, noninvasive procedure.
- The analysis of the research prompted a decision to conduct an evaluation research study on the practice change.

Step 4. Design practice change
- Practice change documents were developed based on the synthesis of the literature.
- Documents were approved, which included: Bladder Scanning Policy and Protocol, UTI Risk Assessment Tool, and Bladder Scanner Information Sheet.
- Inservice education was provided.

Step 5. Implement and evaluate change in practice
- Eight units included in the study were medical-surgical floors, which included step-down units.

Figure 3-12   Application of the model for change to evidence-based practice: evaluation of a bladder scanner protocol implementation: process and outcomes by the Medical-Surgical Research Utilization Team (MSRUT) at West Virginia University Hospitals.

- Low scores on the process indicators demonstrated that the implementation or marketing of the plan during the pilot was not sufficient to affect change and outcome indicators.
- The MSRUT reevaluated the bladder scanner documents and implemented a new plan.
- The MSRUT decided to develop a unit-specific "Change Champion" and involve the unit managers for the next pilot to help with daily follow-up to improve nursing compliance with the new Bladder Scanner Protocol.

Step 6. Integrate and maintain change in practice
- The MSRUT and unit-based practice team members from all participating units revised the existing protocol, improved the paperwork process and revised the Bladder Scanner Marketing Plan.
- By eliminating forms to be completed, nursing compliance has improved.
- Purchase of additional bladder scanners to serve more units is needed because of the high demand for the device.

Figure 3-12   (*Continued*)

patients after discharge, and improving CHF patients' knowledge of self-care. The external data further justified this clinical problem as the focus for an EBP project. The team would probably judge that the initial statement of the clinical problem was sufficiently descriptive.

In the process of collecting internal data and comparing them with external data, the team may fail to find evidence to support the clinical problem as the focus of an EBP project. In that case, the team would discard that clinical problem and search for evidence supporting pursuit of a project on the clinical topic with the second-highest number of votes. In the multivoting example (Figures 3-3 and 3-4), that was nighttime falls by elderly patients due to "sundowner's" syndrome and toileting needs. Alternatively, the team may choose to repeat the multivoting or even repeat the brainstorming process if new ideas have emerged during Step 1. When team members have agreed about a statement of the clinical problem, they are ready to select the patient outcomes and possible interventions to use in conducting the literature search.

CASE 3-3 *One Hospital's Experience*

At WVUH, after the first project on sterile vs. clean gloves was completed, five teams were chartered. They were called research utilization (RU) teams to avoid confusion with the existing practice teams; however, the source of evidence used by the RU teams has been more inclusive than just research. Of these first five teams, three concluded their project at the end of Step 3. One reason was that there was insufficient evidence to support a practice change. Another reason, for at least one team, was that the team represented too diverse a group of clinical specialties to lead to selection of a highly focused clinical problem. The two teams that led to actual practice change represented one clinical specialty each. Subsequently, the teams were reorganized, with nine teams with less diverse clinical interests being created. Additionally, teams were encouraged to select a topic for which there was sufficient evidence to warrant a practice change. For this reason, a team may conduct activities in all of the first three steps of the model before finalizing the selection of the clinical problem that will be the focus of the project. Application of the EBP model in one project is summarized in Figure 3-12.[15] Internal evidence justified a project focused on frequent urinary tract infection.

LINK PROBLEM, INTERVENTIONS, AND OUTCOMES

Use Standardized Classification Systems and Language

The evidence-based practice (EBP) team links the problem statement written earlier with the desired outcomes and potential interventions to develop a specific goal for the EBP project. The steps of the nursing process have been used for decades to guide the care of individual patients. Elements of the nursing process (nursing diagnosis, interventions, and outcomes) can be used to express the goal for an EBP project. While this is a logical framework to use for stating the goal because of nurses' familiarity with the nursing process, its use is not essential to successfully applying the model for EBP change. In fact, many teams have applied the model without using the framework of the nursing process. This chapter will emphasize linking the nursing diagnosis with interventions and outcomes. Alternative approaches will then be briefly discussed.

For at least four decades, nurses have been taught to plan and manage their care of patients using the nursing process. Considerable research to standardize the nursing process language has resulted in several classification systems, including

- Nursing Diagnoses Classification by the North American Nursing Diagnoses Association (NANDA)[16]
- Nursing Interventions Classification (NIC)[17]
- Nursing Outcomes Classification (NOC)[18,19]
- Omaha System[20–22]
- Home Health Care Classification[23]
- Perioperative Nursing Data Set[24]
- Patient Care Data Set[25]
- International Classification of Nursing Practice[26,27]

These classifications are far from static, as research and development continues to make them increasingly useful to practicing nurses. Their intent is to provide language that is nurse-sensitive, meaning that it is relevant to care provided by nurses. The rationale for using standardized languages in practice includes the following:

- Enhance communication about care using terms understood by other nurses.
- Organize and expand knowledge about care.
- Link knowledge with clinical decisions.
- Evaluate the effectiveness of care.
- Identify the needed resources.
- Analyze the costs of care.
- Promote communication among providers across organizations.
- Develop data sets for computerized information systems.

Standardized language also provides a framework for specifically conceptualizing the goal of an EBP project focused on a cohort of patients. Reflecting on the problem statement written earlier, the team would consult the classifications, first selecting the nursing diagnosis that was most relevant to the problem. For instance, in an EBP project focused on reducing the adverse effects of acute confusion in hospitalized older adults,[28] the NANDA nursing diagnosis chosen was "acute confusion." There are 188 nursing diagnoses in the current version of NANDA.[16] For each nursing diagnosis, NANDA presents a definition, defining characteristics, and related factors. This information helps the team select the most appropriate nursing diagnosis for the clinical problem. In the case of "confusion," it helps the team determine if the problem pertains to acute confusion or chronic confusion.

Acute confusion is defined as

- Abrupt onset of reversible disturbances of consciousness, attention, cognition, and perception that develop over a short period of time.[16, p. 41]

In contrast, chronic confusion is defined as

- Irreversible, long-standing, and/or progressive deterioration of intellect and personality characterized by decreased ability to interpret environmental stimuli; decreased capacity for intellectual thought processes; and manifested by disturbances of memory, orientation, and behavior.[16, p. 42]

The precision of these definitions facilitates the decision concerning which to use. Review of the defining characteristics and related factors contributes to the decision.

Some of the defining characteristics of *acute confusion* are[16, p. 41]

- Fluctuation in cognition
- Hallucinations
- Increased agitation
- Lack of motivation to initiate purposeful behavior

Some of the related factors for *acute confusion* are[16, p. 41]

- Over 60 years of age
- Alcohol
- Drug abuse
- Delirium

In contrast, some of the defining characteristics of *chronic confusion* are[16, p. 42]

- Clinical evidence of organic impairment
- Impaired socialization
- Impaired long-term memory
- Impaired short-term memory

Some of the related factors for *chronic confusion* are[16, p. 42]

- Alzheimer disease
- Head injury
- Cerebral vascular attack

The defining characteristics indicate that acute confusion is transitory and reversible, in contrast to chronic confusion. Acute confusion is not an uncommon occurrence when cognitively intact older adults are hospitalized. Research has demonstrated that interventions can be effective in preventing the development of acute confusion during hospitalization. The challenge to nurses is to implement these research-based interventions as a standard of care.

Identify Potential Interventions

Once the team has selected the nursing diagnosis most appropriate for the clinical problem, the next task is to select tentative nursing interventions. Each of the 514 interventions in the 2004 edition of NIC has a definition and assorted activities. Conveniently, one section of the classification links the NANDA nursing diagnoses with potentially relevant nursing interventions.[18]

In the acute confusion project,[28] the nurses selected the NIC intervention "delirium management." The definition of delirium management is

- The provision of a safe and therapeutic environment for the patient who is experiencing an acute confusional state.[18, pp. 275-6]

Under delirium management, there are 36 activities from which to choose. Some of the activities are

- Identify etiological factors causing delirium.
- Monitor neurological status on an ongoing basis.
- Allow the patient to maintain rituals that limit anxiety.
- Provide the patient with information about what is happening and what can be expected to occur in the future.
- Maintain a hazard-free environment.
- Use environmental cues, such as clocks, calendars, and signs.
- Encourage the use of aids that increase sensory input, such as glasses, hearing aids, and dentures.

Research has supported the inclusion of the activities under each NIC intervention. Still, the team members should consider the selected activities tentative until they review and synthesize the evidence during Step 3.

Select Outcome Indicators

Having selected the nursing diagnosis and tentative interventions, the team should then select the target outcomes to be achieved by the end of the EBP project. Outcomes can be patient, health-care system, or financial outcomes. At the least, the EBP project should aim to achieve a patient outcome that would matter to the patient. This is the primary outcome of interest for the EBP project. A common shortcoming during the activities of this step is choosing *making a practice change* as the outcome. Making a practice change is a process and is essential for achieving the patient outcome and other outcomes. As such, it can be considered an intermediate outcome, but the major focus should be on achieving the patient outcome.

To select the patient outcome that the EBP project aims to achieve, the team reviews the selected nursing diagnosis, tentative interventions, and outcome choices in a standardized nursing outcomes classification. In the acute confusion project,[28] the nurses selected the NOC outcome "cognitive orientation." There are 260 outcomes in NOC. Each NOC outcome includes a label, a definition, and an instrument with indicators for achieving the outcome and a rating scale for scoring each indicator. The instrument is a powerful resource for the team to use later, when evaluating the outcome before and after making a practice change, especially if no other instrument for evaluating that particular outcome exists. Conveniently, one section of the classification links the NANDA nursing diagnoses with potentially relevant nursing outcomes.[18]

The definition for the NOC outcome cognitive orientation is

- Ability to identify person, place, and time[18, p. 172]

The instrument for assessing cognitive orientation has seven indicators. It has a five-point Likert-type response scale, with 1 = never demonstrated and 5 = consistently demonstrated. Sample indicators in this scale are[18, p. 172]

- Identifies self
- Identifies current place
- Identifies correct year

After selecting the patient outcome, the team should consider the inclusion of relevant system and financial outcomes. These additional outcomes could pertain to some of the data that were used in justifying the selection of the clinical problem as the project focus. For instance, complaints from patients, families, staff, and other disciplines may have provided the impetus for topic selection, and an outcome might be to reduce the number of such complaints. Data may have indicated that patients classified in one diagnostic related group (DRG) were remaining hospitalized longer than the reimbursable time because of complications of the clinical problem. A relevant outcome could be to reduce the average length of stay so that it does not exceed the reimbursable time. Such an outcome is not trivial to hospital leaders because the hospital is not reimbursed for costs associated with the extra days of hospitalization.

Another possibility is that the data obtained earlier in Step 1 may have demonstrated that the nurses had limited knowledge about the clinical problem or the best evidence for managing the clinical problem. This was the case in the acute confusion project,[28] prompting the setting of an outcome of increasing nurses' scores on a knowledge test after they completed an educational session about acute confusion and delirium management.

Develop a Specific Goal for the EBP Project

Having selected the nursing diagnosis, tentative interventions, and outcomes, the team should write a concise statement linking them. This statement becomes the goal for the EBP project. It will guide the literature search in Step 3. The team should also read the goal statement at the beginning of each team meeting to reaffirm the purpose of the project. For many EBP projects, there will be a vast array of evidence, much of which is tangential to achieving the patient outcome. Without periodically reviewing the goal statement, it can be easy for the team to get off track, prolonging progression through the steps of the model.

Two goal statements for the acute confusion project follow:

- To *achieve* cognitive orientation (outcome) in older patients with acute confusion (nursing diagnosis), we will implement a practice protocol that incorporates delirium management (nursing intervention).

- To *maintain* cognitive orientation (outcome) in older adult patients *at risk of* acute confusion (nursing diagnosis), we will implement a practice protocol that incorporates delirium management (nursing intervention).

Both goal statements are appropriate for acute confusion because, in many instances, older adults do not have acute confusion upon admission to the hospital. However, as older adults, they are at risk of developing acute confusion because of being away from their usual home environment and patterns of daily living. Using both goals guides the EBP team in addressing the needs of both patients who are at risk of acute confusion and those who actually develop acute confusion.

 CASE 3-2.D *Chronic Heart Failure*

Selecting the Nursing Diagnosis

For the fabricated case on chronic heart failure (CHF), the problem statement was "unplanned readmission of CHF patients less than 30 days after discharge due to inadequate self-care." Such readmissions are costly to a hospital because the costs associated with being hospitalized again are not reimbursable. One of the team's goals was to reduce the number of unplanned readmissions less than 30 days after discharge. To accomplish that, the team had to set a goal to address "inadequate self-care." Examination of the NANDA classification revealed two possible nursing diagnoses: knowledge deficit and ineffective therapeutic regimen management. The team chose to set a goal addressing each of these two nursing diagnoses because addressing the knowledge deficit alone does not deal with other reasons why patients are unsuccessful in managing their CHF. Below is a discussion of knowledge deficit and related nursing interventions and outcomes. Following that is a case application of these standardized terms.

The definition of knowledge deficit is[16, p. 130]

- Absence or deficiency of cognitive information related to a specific topic.

The defining characteristics include

- Inaccurate follow-through of instruction
- Verbalization of the problem

Related factors include

- Lack of exposure
- Lack of recall
- Information misinterpretation

Selecting the Nursing Intervention

Reviewing the 29 nursing interventions linked to knowledge deficit, the EBP team selected "disease process teaching."

The definition of disease process teaching is[17, p. 699]

* Assisting the patient to understand information related to a specific disease process.

A few of the 26 activities under disease process teaching include these chosen by the EBP team:

* Appraise the patient's current level of knowledge related to the specific disease process.
* Discuss lifestyle changes that may be required to prevent future complications and/or control the disease process.
* Describe the rationale behind management/therapy/ treatment recommendations.
* Instruct the patient on which signs and symptoms to report to the health-care provider.

Selecting the Nursing Outcomes

Reviewing the 25 outcomes linked to the NANDA nursing diagnosis "knowledge deficit" and the nursing intervention "disease process teaching," the EBP team chose the NOC outcome "treatment regimen knowledge." The definition of treatment regimen knowledge is

* Extent of understanding conveyed about a specific treatment regimen

The instrument for assessing treatment regimen knowledge has 14 indicators. It has a five-point Likert-type response scale, with 1 = none and 5 = extensive. Sample indicators in this scale are

* Description of self-care responsibilities for ongoing treatment
* Description of self-care responsibilities for emergency situations
* Description of prescribed diet
* Description of prescribed medication
* Performance of self-monitoring techniques

Specific Goal for the CHF EBP Project

* To improve treatment regimen knowledge (outcome) for CHF patients with knowledge deficit (nursing diagnosis), we will implement a protocol for disease process teaching about CHF (nursing intervention).

Note that the goal statements for both acute confusion and CHF contain a nursing diagnosis, nursing intervention, and nursing outcome. These terms will be useful in starting the search for evidence in Step 2. During Step 2, the team is likely to locate evidence about more specific nursing interventions relevant to the clinical problem than the general activities listed in NIC. Likewise, the team may locate an instrument that is more specifically designed to measure achievement of the outcome than the more general set of indicators listed for the NOC outcome. The EBP team would decide in Step 3 what the most appropriate nursing interventions are based on its review of the evidence. In Step 4, when planning the practice change, the team would decide which instruments are most appropriate for measuring the patient outcomes.

Setting EBP Project Goal without Using Standardized Language

Informal use of the nursing process

Many EBP teams have applied the model for EBP change without use of the standardized languages. Some of those teams did link the problem, which was not necessarily stated as a nursing diagnosis, with interventions and outcomes, without referring to the classifications. Reasons for not using the standardized languages include

- Nurses were unfamiliar with their existence and purposes.
- Nurse leaders did not require their use in care planning.
- Nurses had difficulty reconciling their use in an interdisciplinary environment.
- Hospital nurses may find it cumbersome to refer to the three most frequently used classifications (NANDA, NIC, and NOC).

These languages are nurse-sensitive, but many of the diagnoses, interventions, and outcomes are relevant to the practices of other health-care disciplines.[29] Increasingly, computerized information systems are integrating the standardized languages into their care planning modules.[23,29–36] This will simplify the use of standardized languages in patient care planning and documentation and create opportunities for nurses to use the data for quality improvement and research purposes. Such computerized information systems potentially will accelerate the adoption of research findings into practice.

Asking answerable questions

Another approach, focused on "asking answerable questions," was developed for use by physicians pursuing evidence-based medicine.[37] This approach has been adopted by some nurses as well.[38] This approach is referred to as asking the PICO question, which has these components:

- **P**   The patient and/or problem of interest
- **I**   The main intervention
- **C**   Comparison intervention(s), if any
- **O**   The clinical outcome of interest

Note the shared elements with the nursing process (interventions and outcomes). The patient or problem of interest may be stated in terms of a medical diagnosis or a clinical problem. The unique feature is the inclusion of a comparison intervention. Following is an application of the PICO question to the CHF case.

 CASE 3-2.E *Chronic Heart Failure*

Elements of the PICO question:

- **P**   Chronic heart failure patients with unplanned readmission in less that 30 days due to inadequate self-care
- **I**   Patient teaching of self-care by staff nurse
- **C**   Long-term management by nurse practitioner via telephone
- **O**   10 percent reduction in unplanned readmissions within 30 days of discharge

PICO question for CHF:

In CHF patients with unplanned readmission in less that 30 days due to inadequate self-care, will long-term management by a nurse practitioner via telephone be more effective than patient teaching of self-care by a staff nurse in reducing the number of unplanned readmissions within 30 days of discharge by 10 percent?

Clearly, using the PICO question approach can help the EBP team have structure for conducting its search for evidence and for setting a target goal to achieve. However, the language may not be as precise as when using the standardized nursing languages. Furthermore, some terms may not have shared meanings among nurses. Once the EBP team has set its goal for the project or written a PICO question, it moves to Step 2 to locate the evidence. First, the team should review its timeline and make any adjustments suggested by the actual length of time consumed by Step 1.

REFERENCES

1. St. Clair K, Larrabee JH. Clean vs. sterile gloves: Which to use for postoperative dressing changes? *Outcomes Manage.* 2002;6(1):17–21.
2. Fanning MF. Reducing postoperative pulmonary complications in cardiac surgery patients with the use of the best evidence. *J Nurs Care Qual.* Apr–Jun 2004;19(2):95–99.
3. Brassard MRD. *The Memory Jogger II: A Pocket Guide of Tools for Continuous Improvement & Effective Planning*, 1st ed. Methuen, MA: GOAL/QPC; 1994.
4. The Joint Commission. *Comprehensive Accreditation Manual for Hospitals: The Official Handbook.* Oakbrook Terrace, IL: The Joint Commission; 2008.
5. Rumsey DJ. *Statistics for Dummies.* Hoboken, NJ: Wiley; 2003.
6. Gonick L, Smith W. *The Cartoon Guide to Statistics.* New York: HarperPerennial; 1993.
7. George ML, Rowlands D, Price M, Maxey J. *The Lean Six Sigma Pocket Toolbook.* New York: McGraw-Hill; 2005.
8. Brassard M. *The Six Sigma Memory Jogger II: A Pocket Guide of Tools for Six Sigma Improvement Teams*, 1st ed. Salem, NH: GOAL/QPC; 2002.
9. The Joint Commission. Performance measurement initiatives. http://www.jointcommission.org/PerformanceMeasurement/PerformanceMeasurement/. Accessed March 7, 2007.

10. Centers for Medicare and Medicaid. Quality initiatives. http://www.cms.hhs.gov/QualityInitiativesGenInfo/. Accessed March 7, 2007.

11. Centers for Medicare and Medicaid. Home health compare. http://www.medicare.gov/HHCompare/Home.asp?version=default &browser=IE%7C7%7CWinXP&language=English& defaultstatus=0&pagelist=Home&CookiesEnabledStatus= True. Accessed March 7, 2007.

12. Centers for Medicare and Medicaid. Hospital compare. http://www.hospitalcompare.hhs.gov/Hospital/Search/SearchCriteria. asp?version=default&browser=IE%7C7%7CWinXP& language=English&defaultstatus=0&pagelist=Home. Accessed March 7, 2007.

13. American Nurses Association. National Center for Nursing Quality. http://www.nursingquality.org/. Accessed March 7, 2007.

14. University HealthSystem Consortium. Home page. http://www.uhc.edu/home.asp. Accessed March 7, 2007.

15. Daniels C, Medical-Surgical Research Utilization Team (MSRUT). Application of the model for change to evidence-based practice: Evaluation of a bladder scanner protocol implementation: Process and outcomes. Morgantown, WV: West Virginia University Hospitals; 2007.

16. NANDA International. *Nursing Diagnoses: Definitions and Classification 2007–2008*. Philadelphia, PA: NANDA International; 2007.

17. Dochterman JM, Bulechek GM. *Nursing Interventions Classification (NIC)*. St. Louis, MO: Elsevier Mosby, Inc.; 2004.

18. Moorhead S, Johnson M, Maas M. *Iowa Outcomes Project: Nursing Outcomes Classification (NOC)*. St. Louis, MO: Elsevier Mosby, Inc.; 2004.

19. Moorhead S, Johnson M, Maas M, Reed D. Testing the nursing outcomes classification in three clinical units in a community hospital. *J Nurs Meas*. Fall 2003;11(2):171–181.

20. Bowles KH, Martin KS. Three decades of Omaha System research: Providing the map to discover new directions. *Stud Health Technol Inform*. 2006;122:994.

21. Martin KS, Elfrink VL, Monsen KA, Bowles KH. Introducing standardized terminologies to nurses: Magic wands and other strategies. *Stud Health Technol Inform*. 2006;122:596–599.
22. Martin KS, Norris J. The Omaha System: A model for describing practice. *Holist Nurs Pract*. Oct 1996;11(1):75–83.
23. Saba VK. Nursing classifications: Home Health Care Classification System (HHCC): An overview. *Online J Issues Nurs*. 2002;7(3):9. http://www.nursingworld.org/MainMenu Categories/ANAMarketplace/ANAPeriodicals/OJIN/TableofCon tents/Vol31998/Vol3No21998/HHCC AnOverview.aspx.
24. American Perioperative Registered Nurses. Perioperative Nursing Data Set.http://www.aorn.org/PracticeResources/PNDS/. Accessed July 11, 2007.
25. Ozbolt JG, Fruchtnicht JN, Hayden JR. Toward data standards for clinical nursing information. *JAMIA*. 1994;1(2):175–185.
26. Hyun S, Park HA. Cross-mapping the ICNP with NANDA, HHCC, Omaha System and NIC for unified nursing language system development. International Classification for Nursing Practice. International Council of Nurses. North American Nursing Diagnosis Association. Home Health Care Classification. Nursing Interventions Classification. *Int Nurs Rev*. Jun 2002;49(2):99–110.
27. International Council of Nurses. International Classification of Nursing Practice. http://www.icn.ch/icnp.htm. Accessed April 18, 2007.
28. Rosswurm MA, Larrabee JH. A model for change to evidence-based practice. *Image J Nurs Sch*. 1999;31(4):317–322.
29. Smith K, Smith V. Successful interdisciplinary documentation through nursing interventions classification. *Semin Nurse Manag*. Jun 2002;10(2):100–104.
30. Larrabee JH, Boldreghini S, Elder-Sorrells K, et al. Evaluation of documentation before and after implementation of a nursing information system in an acute care hospital. *Comput Nurs*. Mar–Apr 2001;19(2):56–65; quiz 66-58.
31. Keenan G, Yakel E, Marriott D. HANDS: A revitalized technology supported care planning method to improve nursing handoffs. *Stud Health Technol Inform*. 2006;122:580–584.

32. Delaney C, Mehmert PA, Prophet C, et al. Standardized nursing language for healthcare information systems. *J Med Syst.* Aug 1992;16(4):145–159.

33. Brooks BA, Massanari K. Implementation of NANDA nursing diagnoses online. North American Nursing Diagnosis Association. *Comput Nurs.* Nov–Dec 1998;16(6):320–326.

34. Prophet CM. The evolution of a clinical database: From local to standardized clinical languages. *Proc AMIA Symp.* 2000:660–664.

35. Allred SK, Smith KF, Flowers L. Electronic implementation of national nursing standards—NANDA, NOC and NIC as an effective teaching tool. *J Healthc Inf Manag.* Fall 2004; 18(4):56–60.

36. Flo K. Nursing documentation with NANDA and NIC in a comprehensive HIS/EPR system. *Stud Health Technol Inform.* 2006;122:1009.

37. Sackett DL. Evidence-based medicine: how to practice and teach EBM. 2nd ed. Edinburgh: Churchill Livingstone; 2000.

38. Melnyk BM, Fineout-Overholt E. *Evidence-Based Practice in Nursing & Healthcare: A Guide to Best Practice.* Philadelphia: Lippincott Williams & Wilkins; 2005.

39. Sparks A, Boyer D, Gambrel A, et al. The clinical benefits of the bladder scanner: A research synthesis. *J Nurs Care Qual.* Jul–Sep 2004;19(3):188–192.

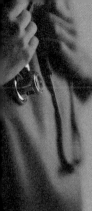

Chapter 4

STEP 2: LOCATE THE BEST EVIDENCE

- ■ **IDENTIFY TYPES AND SOURCES OF EVIDENCE**
  - — Clinical Practice Guidelines
  - — Systematic Reviews
  - — Research
    - ■ *Critical appraisal topics (CATs)*
  - — Expert Committee Reports

- ■ **REVIEW RESEARCH CONCEPTS**
  - — Quantitative Research
    - ■ *Introduction*
    - ■ *Internal validity*
      - ○ *Threats to internal validity*
    - ■ *External validity*
    - ■ *Research designs*
  - — Qualitative Research
    - ■ *Introduction*
    - ■ *Qualitative research traditions*
    - ■ *Analysis*
    - ■ *Trustworthiness*
      - ○ *Credibility*
      - ○ *Dependability*
      - ○ *Confirmability*
      - ○ *Transferability*
    - ■ *Contributions of qualitative research to evidence-based practice*

■ **PLAN THE SEARCH AND REVIEW**
   — Guidelines for Conducting a Systematic Review
     ▪ *Research question*
     ▪ *Search strategy*
     ▪ *Inclusion criteria*
     ▪ *Critical appraisal*
       ○ *Choose or develop critical appraisal tools for different types of evidence*
       ○ *Choose or design an evidence table template for displaying data about research evidence*
     ▪ *Synthesis*

■ **CONDUCT THE SEARCH**
   — *Learning to Search Using Electronic Databases*
   — *Tips for Searching for the Evidence*
   — *Examples of Searching for Evidence*

IDENTIFY TYPES AND SOURCES OF EVIDENCE

In this step, the evidence-based practice (EBP) team locates the best evidence available that is relevant to the project's goal. Types of evidence include clinical practice guidelines (CPG), systematic reviews, research reports, and expert committee reports. These types of evidence produce evidence for practice that varies in quality and credibility. An exemplary hierarchy for strength of evidence appears in Figure 4-1, with evidence being listed in descending order of strength. Systematic reviews, CPG, research reports, and expert committee reports are available in print or on the Internet.

Clinical Practice Guidelines

"Clinical practice guidelines are systematically developed statements to assist practitioner and patient decisions about appropriate health care for specific clinical circumstances."[1, p. 38]

Level	Description*
1a	Systematic review of randomized controlled trials (RCTs) with homogeneity
1b	One properly randomized RCT with narrow confidence interval
1c	Well-designed controlled trials without randomization
2a	Systematic review of cohort studies with homogeneity
2b	One cohort study
3a	Systematic review of case-control studies with homogeneity
3b	One case-control study
4	Descriptive correlational studies, descriptive comparative studies, case series
5	Opinions of respected clinical experts, descriptive studies, case reports, or reports from expert committees

*Based on other levels of evidence hierarchies[9,59]

Figure 4-1   Hierarchy of evidence for practice.

A CPG is a document that presents recommendations for practice based on systematic reviews of available evidence. Usually, a CPG is developed by a collaborative panel of content experts who prepare evidence tables and rate each recommendation based on the strength of the evidence. The intent in developing a CPG is to give providers information for clinical decision making through education and continuing education.[2]

The EBP team should consider searching for a CPG that is relevant to its project before searching for research reports. If the team finds a relevant CPG, the time needed for critiquing and synthesizing the evidence will be reduced. The team could limit searching for other forms of evidence to the years since the CPG was published or released. There are a number of Internet sources for CPGs (see Appendix A).

The National Guideline Clearinghouse™ (NGC) is a freely accessible database of evidence-based CPG. NGC operates under the auspices of the Agency for Healthcare Research and Quality, U.S. Department of Health and Human Services. The contents of NGC include

• Summaries of the guidelines and their development.
• Links to full-text guidelines or ordering information for print copies.
• Palm PDA downloads of the NGC guideline summary.

Because a guideline located via NGC is a summary and not necessarily the full text, EBP team members may need to access the full-text guideline before critically appraising the CPG.

Specific sites for accessing nursing best practice guidelines include

• **Registered Nurses Association of Ontario—Best Practice Guidelines available for purchase:**

— http://www.rnao.org/bestpractices/index.asp

• **JBI ConNect by Joanna Briggs Institute for Evidence Based Nursing and Midwifery—subscription fee:**

— http://www.jbiconnect.org/index.php

• **University of Iowa Gerontological Nursing Interventions Research Center—guidelines available for purchase:**

— http://www.nursing.uiowa.edu/consumers_patients/evidence_based.htm

• **Association of Women's Health, Obstetric, and Neonatal Nurses (AWHONN) Standards and Guidelines—available for purchase:**

— http://www.awhonn.org/awhonn/

• **Emergency Nursing World:**

— http://www.enw.org/TOC.htm

• **American Association of periOperative Nurses—Practice Resources available for purchase:**

— http://www.aorn.org/

- **McGill University Health Centre—links to guidelines:**
  — http://muhc-ebn.mcgill.ca/index.html

Systematic Reviews

A systematic review is a critical analysis, using a rigorous methodology, of original research identified by a comprehensive search of the literature. A systematic review presents conclusions about the current best evidence on a topic. A meta-analysis, a type of systematic review, "is the statistical combination of at least two studies to produce a single estimate of the effect of the health care intervention under consideration."[3, p. 700]

There are increasing numbers of systematic reviews available. The advantages of systematic reviews for nurses are that they provide information about the best evidence and its generalizability, or its applicability to diverse settings.[4] The use of systematic reviews reduces the time needed to make the EBP change because the team does not have to search for, critically appraise, and synthesize all of the research evidence. The team can limit searching for other forms of evidence to the years since the systematic review was published or released.

The EBP team should consider searching for systematic reviews before searching for original research. Currently, the largest database of systematic reviews is the Cochrane Library, developed by the Cochrane Collaboration, which was founded in 1993. It generates and disseminates systematic reviews of the effectiveness of health-care interventions.[5] Some health-care organizations subscribe to the Cochrane Library or have access to it through affiliation with a university. Otherwise, a review can be purchased from the Cochrane Library by clicking on the link to the PDF copy of the desired systematic review and following the instructions. The Cochrane Library can be accessed at http://www.cochrane.org/index.htm.

The Campbell Collaboration, initiated in 2000, generates and disseminates systematic reviews of the effectiveness of interventions in the social, behavioral, and educational fields.[6]

Systematic reviews can be purchased at http://www.campbell-collaboration.org/.

Other databases for systematic reviews are also available online (see Appendix B).

Research

Research is rigorous, systematic investigation to further develop existing knowledge and to generate new knowledge to inform practice. Electronic resources make searching for research reports more manageable, efficient, and thorough than in the past, when hard-copy indexes were the best resource. Some electronic resources are free, while some require a fee for use. Accessing any of them requires a computer with Internet access and a Web browser. Some databases for searching are free (see Appendix C), and others require a subscription (see Appendix D). The EBP team will be able to access those to which its health-care organization or affiliated university subscribes.

The EBP team should consider starting its search for research reports by searching PubMed. It indexes a large number of journals, and its use is free. PubMed and Cumulative Index of Nursing and Allied Health Literature (CINAHL) each index some journals that the other bibliographic database does not. Therefore, the team should also search CINAHL, if it is accessible. If other relevant databases are accessible, the team should consider searching those as well so that it can be confident that its search was comprehensive.

Critical appraisal topics (CATs)

A CAT is a structured abstract of a medical journal article.[7] Some are published in the scientific literature. Some are available online. The EBP team may decide to include CATs as evidence for its project. However, the team should also perform a critical appraisal of the original research reports to form its own judgments about the research. CATs can be accessed online (see Appendix E).

Expert Committee Reports

The last type of evidence to consider is expert committee reports, which are consensus statements based primarily on the clinical expertise of the committee members. Some expert committee reports may also be based on scientific evidence. In addition to being called expert committee reports and consensus statements, they may be called position statements or standards of practice, especially when issued by nursing organizations.

 CASE 4-1 *Example of a Consensus Statement on Chronic Heart Failure*

A panel of experts of the Association of Palliative Medicine Science Committee reviewed the evidence about the effectiveness of using oxygen for the relief of breathlessness in chronic obstructive pulmonary disease (COPD), advanced cancer, and chronic heart failure (CHF). Very few RCTs were located. There were no relevant studies for CHF and few for advanced cancer. There were RCTs on the use of oxygen in COPD, but few of them evaluated reduction of breathlessness as an outcome measure. Recommendations were based on available existing evidence and expert opinion, including that of the Royal College of Physicians report.[8]

Some expert committee reports are developed using a structured methodology. For instance, these are the steps in the process used by the National Institutes of Health (NIH) Consensus Development Program:

1. An independent expert panel is assembled.
2. Four to six questions on the efficacy, risks, and clinical applications of a technology and one on directions for future research are the focus of a consensus conference.
3. A systematic literature review pertinent to the questions is prepared by one of the Evidence-Based Practice Centers in the Agency for Healthcare Research and Quality for use by the panel.

4. Invited experts present data to the panel in public sessions, followed by discussion. Then the panel prepares
the consensus statement during executive session.
5. Next, the draft conference statement is presented in a ple-
nary session, followed by public discussion. The final statement is posted on the web site http://consensus.nih.gov.

The EBP team should consider searching for expert committee reports if, after a comprehensive search for CPG, systematic
reviews, and research reports, it has found little or no evidence
relevant to its topic. Expert committee reports can be located
on professional web sites and in the literature. Nursing position
statements or standards of practice are available online (see
Appendix F).

Some web sites of professional organizations may not post
position statements or standards of practice. Of those that do,
some have a link on the home page labeled "position statements" or "standards of practice." On other sites, the team will
have to search, if a search feature is available.

Many expert committee reports are published. Therefore,
searching the electronic databases will identify any expert committee reports that are relevant to the EBP team's topic. Another
way to locate expert committee reports is to conduct a browser
search using a search engine such as Google or Yahoo and
including the keywords "expert committee report," "consensus
statement," "standards of practice," or "position statements."
One caution about searching for evidence on the World Wide
Web: the hits may not be based on scientific evidence. Also,
there are likely to be many hits that duplicate those obtained by
searching the electronic databases or government and professional web sites. For instance, in a Google search using "expert
committee report" and "chronic heart failure," there were hun-
dreds of hits. All the hits on the first few pages were for published articles, indicating that they could have been located by
searching electronic databases.

There will be some clinical problems for which a systematic
review or CPG is not available. Therefore, members of the EBP

team need to learn or review key information about research and how to critically appraise it.

REVIEW RESEARCH CONCEPTS

To perform a critical appraisal, the EBP team members need to understand the different research designs and the factors that influence which designs produce the best evidence of the effectiveness of an intervention. Research can be classified as being either quantitative or qualitative. Following is a general introduction to basic concepts in research. Because the majority of the evidence on intervention effectiveness is produced by quantitative research, the emphasis will be on quantitative research.

Quantitative Research

Introduction

The purpose of quantitative research, depending on the question of interest and the design of the research, is to describe a concept in depth, present data about the incidence of a health problem or complication, identify associations among variables, examine differences between groups or times, identify predictors of an outcome, and evaluate the effectiveness of an intervention. Examples of research questions for which quantitative research is the appropriate investigative approach include

- What is self-care for patients with CHF?
- What percentage of this hospital's annual census has CHF?
- What is the relationship between self-care and unexpected hospitalization of patients with CHF?
- Are there differences in the number of unexpected hospitalizations between a group of CHF patients who receive usual care and a group of CHF patients who receive long-term disease management by a specialized nurse practitioner?
- What are the predictors of unplanned hospitalization for CHF management?

• How effective is an intervention consisting of long-term disease management by a specialized nurse practitioner in reducing hospitalizations and mortality?

To answer these types of questions, quantitative research

• Relies on statistical analysis of *numbers* that represent scores for measured concepts.

• Relies on measuring concepts with instruments, either physiological or attitudinal.

• Refers to measured concepts as variables. The most basic categories of variables are

— Dependent or outcome: variables that you want to influence.

— Independent: variables that are intended or thought to produce a change in the dependent variable.

▪ An intervention is a type of independent variable.

— Extraneous or confounding: variables other than the independent variable that can influence the dependent variable or the independent variable, confounding the interpretation of results.

• Relies on a sufficient number of participants to have enough power to identify the effectiveness of an intervention or the relationships among variables.

— A larger sample size is more representative of the population being sampled.

— The effect size is the strength of the relationship between variables and can vary from very small to large.

— The power to detect the effect of an intervention is dependent on how large the effect size is and the number of participants.

— The smaller the effect size to be detected, the larger the sample that is needed.

— The significance of the effect size or a relationship is statistically calculated.

▪ Significance is reported as a probability or p-value.

▪ The traditional significance level used in most studies is $p < .05$.

■ A $p < .05$ means that only 5 times out of 100 would an effect or relationship be detected by *chance* instead of because a true effect or relationship exists.

Internal validity

For readers to have confidence in the findings of a study, it must have *internal validity*. Internal validity, or the extent to which an inference can be made that the independent variable, such as the intervention, influences the dependent variable, is reliant upon

• Instrument reliability and validity
  — Instrument reliability: the consistency with which the instrument measures the variable.
  — Instrument validity: the degree to which the instrument measures the intended concept.
• The extent to which a study is designed to control for the influence of extraneous variables: the greater this control, the stronger the evidence produced by the study

Weak or questionable internal validity limits the strength of the study's evidence and is a *key concern when critically appraising a research article*.

Threats to internal validity

The strength of the research design is dependent upon how well it controls for the threats to internal validity. There are both external and internal threats to internal validity that must be controlled.

• Controlling *external* threats to internal validity means assuring the constancy of conditions for data collection by the following methods:
  — Constancy of time (time of day or year), if relevant
  — Constancy of intervention implementation
  — Constancy of approach in data collection (use of scripts when recruiting participants or conducting interviews)

Another condition to consider is the use of homogeneous settings to minimize the influence of diversity on the dependent variable. Also, avoid the introduction of other initiatives that could influence the dependent variable.

- Controlling *internal* threats to internal validity means controlling for variability of study participant characteristics (extraneous variables) that could influence the dependent variable. This is done through the sampling plan. The following are examples of sampling plans:
  — Random assignment: controls *all* potentially confounding variables
  — Alternative plans when random assignment is not feasible:
    - Homogeneity: exclude potential participants with a potentially confounding characteristic (e.g., smokers).
    - Blocking: include potentially confounding variables in the design as independent variables, for example, pre-planning a comparison of groups based on differences in a characteristic (smoker vs. nonsmoker).
    - Matching: for each participant in the intervention group, have a participant in the control group (no intervention) that is matched on the basis of all potentially confounding variables, such as gender, age, smoking status, and so on.

External validity

For readers to judge that study findings are applicable to their work site, the study must have *external validity*. External validity or generalizability, meaning the applicability of study findings to other settings and populations beyond the site of the study, is largely dependent on the characteristics of the study's sample and how representative of the general population the participants are.

Research designs

Research designs are either experimental or nonexperimental. Experimental studies are the best designs for investigating the effectiveness of an intervention. These designs have three components:

- An intervention, that is, manipulation of the independent variable
- A control group
- Random *assignment* of participants to the experimental and control groups

The following is a description of research designs in descending order based on the ability to control the internal threats to internal validity.[9,M-21,10]:

- An RCT (experimental design) is considered the "gold standard" for investigating intervention effectiveness.
- Quasi-experimental designs are the second-best designs for investigating the effectiveness of an intervention. The limitation is that they lack random assignment to the experimental and control groups.
- Cohort studies are longitudinal designs that follow a group of people (a cohort), examining how exposure to some suspected risk factor (e.g., smoking) differs within the group to identify whether exposure is likely to cause a specified event (e.g., lung cancer).[11]
- Case control studies are cross-sectional designs that examine a group of people who have experienced an adverse event (e.g., lung cancer) and a group of people who have not experienced the same event to determine how exposure to a suspected risk factor (e.g., smoking) differed between the two groups.[11]
- Descriptive comparative designs compare differences in a variable, either between two or more groups or within one group at different time points. Finding a significant difference between groups or between times does not imply causation.
- Descriptive correlation designs measure at least two variables and evaluate their relationship. Finding a relationship does not imply causation.

- Descriptive exploratory designs measure and describe as few as one variable. This is an appropriate design when the research question is about a concept for which there is little or no descriptive information.

For some EBP team members, this introduction to quantitative research may refresh their memories of knowledge about research; however, for most members, this will be new information. The team members should discuss their need to consult with a nurse researcher to teach and mentor the team about research. Other resources to help the team members develop the skills needed to read and appraise research include journal articles, research textbooks, and research guides. One such research guide by Borbasi, Jackson, and Langford[12] is written for direct-care nurses.

Journal articles have been identified as the primary information source used by nurses.[13] A number of journal articles provide an introduction to research[14] and a "how-to" description on critiquing research.[15–21] A series of 12 journal articles[22–33] discusses separate aspects of research critiques, such as threats to internal validity, how to interpret different statistical tests, and the validity and reliability of measurement instruments. Finally, there are online resources, including tutorials or fact sheets and nursing research courses (see Appendix G).

Qualitative Research

Introduction

The purpose of qualitative research is to study human phenomena using holistic methodologies. For instance, phenomenology describes a phenomenon of interest, grounded theory explains a social process, and ethnography describes a culture. Qualitative research provides in-depth knowledge that is holistic, incorporating contextual influences. End products are either an in-depth or "thick" description of a phenomenon, a model of processes, or a culture.[10,34]

Examples of questions for which qualitative research is the appropriate investigative approach include

- How do CHF patients define self-care?
- What is the "lived" experience of adjusting to having CHF?
- What is the basic social process of being a partner with the provider in long-term management of CHF?
- What is the culture of a CHF clinic like?

In general, qualitative research relies on[34]

- Analysis of text, observations, and artifacts.
- The researcher functioning as the research instrument.
  - This is in contrast to quantitative research, in which the researcher uses objective measurement and statistical analysis.
- Data gathering via informal conversations; loosely guided interviews; review of documents; and examination of artifacts, photographs, video, and other such material.
- Analysis that begins with data from the first participant and is ongoing.
- Adequate selection of participants who can be good informants, meaning that they know about and can talk about what the researcher is investigating.
- Sampling that achieves data saturation, meaning that no new themes emerge when additional participants are added.
  - Interviews tend to start with convenience sampling and, depending on the research question and the research tradition, move on to other sampling strategies.
    - Snowballing is recruiting participants from persons who have already participated.
    - Purposive sampling is deliberately recruiting participants who can provide more in-depth information on some aspect of the evolving description.
    - Other sampling plans are used as appropriate.
    - Sampling ceases when data saturation is reached.

— Sample sizes tend to be smaller than in quantitative research.

  ■ Phenomenology: 10 or less.

  ■ Ethnography and grounded theory: 20–40.

• Writing or typing transcriptions of the interviews; writing memos about the interviews, observations, or examinations of other data sources; and keeping an audit trail of decisions made during the analysis.

Qualitative research traditions

There are a number of qualitative research approaches or traditions. Those most common in the nursing literature are

• Content analysis

  — Purpose: To describe a concept, phenomenon, or event

  — Product: A description

• Grounded theory

  — Purpose: To explore social processes within human interactions

  — Product: Explanations of social processes and structures that are grounded in empirical data

• Phenomenology

  — Purpose: To describe the essence of the lived experience of some aspect of everyday life

  — Product: A "thick" description of the phenomenon

• Ethnography

  — Purpose: To develop theories of culture

  — Product: A factual description and analysis of aspects of the way of life of a particular culture or subculture

Analysis

Analysis in qualitative research, in general, occurs in two phases, referred to as (1) reductionistic and (2) constructionistic.[10,34]

First, in the reductionistic phase, the researcher reads the transcripts and memos and codes segments of those data. Next, the researcher examines the codes, searching for themes and contemplating their conceptual labels. This is, in general, an iterative, not a linear, process, meaning that, in critically considering themes, the researcher constantly moves back and forth between examining themes and examining the codes that suggest them. This is referred to as "constant comparison." Through this process, the themes "emerge."

Second, during the constructionistic phase of analysis, the researcher constructs either an in-depth description of the phenomenon, a model of social processes, or a description of a culture.

Trustworthiness

The notion of trustworthiness is for qualitative research what validity is for quantitative research. Because of the differences between quantitative and qualitative research, the criteria for validity that apply to quantitative research do not apply to qualitative research. One well-accepted approach to evaluating the trustworthiness of qualitative research consists of the following four criteria:[35,36]

- Credibility
- Dependability
- Confirmability
- Transferability

Credibility

Credibility is the qualitative equivalent of internal validity in quantitative research. When critically appraising the credibility of a qualitative research study, one seeks to answer the question: do the findings reflect reality? Credibility depends on many aspects of the study, including how well qualified the researcher is to conduct the study; the extent to which the researcher used an established research tradition; whether or not the sampling plan was appropriate to answer the research question; whether or not the researcher performed "member checks," sharing results and obtaining feedback from some of the participants; and how in-depth the description of the phenomenon, model of social processes, or culture is.

Dependability
Dependability pertains to whether or not the study could be replicated by another researcher. To meet that criterion, the report of the qualitative study must provide a sufficiently detailed description of the research design and the procedures used in collecting and analyzing data, and a critical analysis of the research methodology as it was implemented.

Confirmability
Confirmability is the qualitative equivalent of objectivity in quantitative research and pertains to whether or not the findings reflect the participants' experience and not just the researcher's. To meet this criterion, the report of the qualitative study must provide a sufficiently detailed description of the researcher's own preconceptions and how those influenced decisions throughout the research study.

Transferability
Transferability is the qualitative equivalent of generalizability in quantitative research, meaning that it is the extent to which the findings of the qualitative study can be applicable in other settings. The findings of a qualitative study are highly dependent upon the context in which the study is conducted. Therefore, qualitative researchers rarely make inferences about transferability to other settings.[36] For readers to judge the potential transferability of a qualitative study's findings to their own setting, the research report must have a full description of the contextual factors that influenced the findings.

As with quantitative research, this introduction to qualitative research may refresh the memories of some EBP team members, but, for most members, this may be new information. The team may benefit from teaching and mentoring about qualitative research by a nurse researcher. Other resources to help develop the skills needed in reading[37,38] and appraising qualitative research include journal articles[39–42] and research textbooks and guides, including the one previously mentioned.[12] Educational resources for learning about qualitative research and how to critically appraise qualitative research are available online (Appendix H).

Contributions of qualitative research to evidence-based practice

During the past decade, there has been increasingly persuasive evidence that qualitative research has the potential for making several worthwhile contributions to EBP change.[43–50] A critical analysis of the literature[45] concluded that there were at least five contributions that qualitative research findings made to EBP:

1. Generation of hypotheses

    a. The findings of some qualitative research studies have generated hypotheses for testing in subsequent quantitative research studies.

2. Generation of research questions

    a. The findings of some qualitative research studies and the identification of the remaining gaps in the knowledge base have generated research questions for testing in subsequent quantitative research studies.

3. Development and validation of research instruments

    a. Research instruments with excellent content and construct validity have used qualitative research findings to generate items for the instrument.

4. Design of nursing interventions

    a. Qualitative research findings, either alone or in combination with quantitative research findings, have been used to design nursing interventions for EBP changes.

5. Evaluation of EBP changes

    a. Qualitative research can complement the quantitative evaluation of EBP changes, providing holistic insights that are not available by using quantitative evaluation alone.

    b. The recently developed method of qualitative outcome analysis uses qualitative research findings to design the practice change and, subsequently, uses qualitative research to evaluate patient outcomes.[51]

Recently, there has been increasing emphasis on qualitative researchers producing meta-syntheses of qualitative research studies.[46] Such meta-syntheses will provide direct-care nurses with summaries and recommendations of qualitative research findings, as systematic reviews currently do for quantitative studies.

Also recently, there have been initiatives among qualitative researchers to use meta-syntheses to produce materials that can be used by direct-care nurses to make EBP changes.[49] Such materials will reduce the time required for direct-care nurses to conduct EBP projects.

PLAN THE SEARCH AND REVIEW

To plan the search for evidence, the members of the EBP team must consider how they will use the evidence. For their review of the *research* evidence to be most informative, the team should plan to conduct a systematic review. During the past 20 years, conducting systematic reviews has come to be viewed as a new form of research, as the methodology for conducting systematic reviews has become more rigorous.[52,53] The EBP team must be familiar with the elements of a systematic review to adequately plan the search for evidence.

Guidelines for Conducting a Systematic Review

A number of guidelines for conducting a systematic review have been published.[3,4,53–58] The collective consensus is that the elements of a systematic review include the following, which will be briefly discussed:

1. Research question
2. Search strategy
3. Inclusion criteria
4. Critical appraisal
5. Synthesis

Research question

Conducting a systematic review is a form of research, so it makes sense that the EBP team will need a research question to guide the search for the evidence. If the team members have developed a specific goal for the project using nursing process language in Step 1, they can edit the goal into a question. For example, in Case 3-2.D, the specific goal for the CHF EBP project was:

To improve treatment regimen knowledge (outcome) for CHF patients with knowledge deficit (nursing diagnosis), we will implement a protocol for disease process teaching about CHF (nursing intervention).

This goal statement can be edited into the following question:

Will a protocol for disease process teaching about CHF (nursing intervention) improve treatment regimen knowledge (outcome) for CHF patients with knowledge deficit (nursing diagnosis)?

If the EBP team developed a PICO question during Step 1, that can serve as the research question for the systematic review. For instance, the PICO question in Case 3-2.E was:

In CHF patients with unplanned readmission in less than 30 days due to inadequate self-care, will long-term management by a nurse practitioner via telephone be more effective than patient teaching of self-care by a staff nurse in reducing the number of unplanned readmissions within 30 days of discharge by 10 percent?

Further information about developing the research question to guide the systematic review is available online.[59]

Search strategy

Before starting the search, the EBP team needs to decide what sources of evidence it will search. Selection of databases will, in part, depend upon the databases to which the team members have access. It will also depend on the nature of the clinical problem and whether or not the team has access to a specialty database pertaining to that problem, such as PsycINFO, which indexes literature about psychology.

In addition to deciding which databases to search, the EBP team should plan on examining reference lists of relevant articles, once those are retrieved. This approach may help the team identify additional research studies that were not found while searching electronic databases.

Inclusion criteria

The EBP team should decide on the inclusion criteria for the evidence prior to searching for the evidence. Those criteria should pertain to the patient population, interventions, and outcomes that are addressed in the research question for the review. The criteria should also specify years of publication to be searched, research study designs, geographic location, and type of health-care setting.

The keywords in the research question for the review become the keywords that the EBP team should use when conducting the evidence search. For instance, with the Case 3-2.E CHF example, the team would search for research that studied

- CHF patients
- Long-term management by a nurse practitioner
- Patient teaching of self-care by a direct-care nurse
- The number of unplanned readmissions within 30 days of discharge

In addition to keywords, other inclusion criteria depend on the purpose of the review and should specify

- Years to be searched
  - Five to ten years should be sufficient if the purpose of the review is to determine the effectiveness of an intervention.
  - Articles published more than ten years ago may be included if the purpose of the review is a summary of what is known about the clinical problem.
- Study designs
  - Experimental designs
    - RCTs and quasi-experimental studies are the strongest research designs to evaluate the effectiveness of an intervention (Figure 4-1).
      - The team may plan to use only studies with these designs.
      - Further information about some research designs is available online.[59]
  - Nonexperimental designs
    - The team may need to plan on including studies with these designs if it is unable to locate RCTs and quasi-experimental studies.
      - Cohort designs
      - Case control designs
      - Descriptive comparative designs
      - Descriptive correlation designs
      - Descriptive exploratory designs

The team should consider the added advantage of including qualitative research studies.

- Geographic location of the study sample
  - The team should decide whether or not to specify that the studies included were conducted in a certain type of geographic location, such as

- Urban
- Rural
- National
- International

Limiting the research reports included to those with geographic similarity increases the likelihood that the study findings will be applicable or generalizable to the team's work site. On the other hand, including all relevant research reports, regardless of geography, is more comprehensive. Furthermore, if findings about the effectiveness of an intervention are consistent or homogeneous across the studies, the strength of the evidence is stronger.

- Type of health-care setting
  - The team should decide whether or not to specify that included studies were conducted in a certain type of health-care setting, such as
    - Hospital
      - For-profit, not-for-profit, military, government, or other
      - Academic medical center, community hospital, or other
    - Nursing home
    - Outpatient clinic
    - Patients' homes

Including only studies conducted in settings similar to the EBP team's own health-care setting will provide evidence that is most directly applicable to the EBP team's own health-care setting. However, this choice may also narrow the hits to an insufficient pool of research evidence. The team may decide to add this inclusion criterion only if the number of hits is huge.

The inclusion criteria will help the EBP team screen research reports before starting the critical appraisal. The team should consider having two members independently decide if each study meets the inclusion criteria to avoid selection bias, such as the temptation to include only studies that demonstrated the effectiveness of the intervention and to exclude those that don't.[60]

Critical appraisal

Critical appraisal is systematically analyzing research to evaluate its validity, results, and relevance prior to using it to change practice.[61] When planning the critical appraisal, the EBP team should (1) choose or develop critical appraisal tools for different types of evidence and (2) choose or design an evidence table template for displaying data about all included evidence.

Choose or Develop Critical Appraisal Tools for Different Types of Evidence

The EBP team will benefit later while critically appraising the research evidence if the members choose from among existing critical appraisal tools or develop or modify one for the purposes of collecting the data about and critically appraising each evidence document. A number of critical appraisal tools exist. Some are checklists with questions to guide the appraisal, and others are forms. These tools are designed for appraising CPGs, systematic reviews, and research. Some of the research appraisal tools are for research in general. Others are for specific research designs, including RCTs, cohort studies, and case control studies. Checklists or questionnaires to use while collecting data about a research study have been published in some journal articles discussing literature critique.[17,20,39,62] Examples of existing forms appear in Figures 4-2 to 4-4. Others can also be found in published books[10] and journal articles.[63,64] An example of a checklist for a research study appears in Figure 4-5, and a checklist for systematic reviews appears in Figure 4-6. The team members may wish to examine several checklists before making a choice. They may decide to use one "as is," modify an existing form or checklist, or create one. Tools for critically appraising the different types of evidence are available online (Appendix I).

Citation (authors, year, title of article, journal, volume, issue, pages): _____

Aims, research questions or hypotheses: _____

Type: ____ Quantitative ____ Mixed methods

Study site: _____

Sample: Size ____ Sampling plan ____ Demographics ____

Variables and instruments:

Dependent _____

Independent (including intervention) _____

Potential confounding _____

Design:

Experimental

☐ Randomized controlled trial
☐ Experiment
☐ Quasi-experimental

Nonexperimental

☐ Cohort study
☐ Case control study
☐ Descriptive comparative study
☐ Descriptive correlation study
☐ Descriptive exploratory study

Figure 4-2   Literature review worksheet for quantitative research.

Results: _____

Recommendations: _____

Strengths:

Internal validity _____

External validity _____

Limitations:

Internal validity _____

External validity _____

Analysis

Clinical significance: _____

Credibility of results: _____

Intervention applicable to my setting: _____

Acceptability of benefit vs. risk: _____

Acceptability of costs: _____

Figure 4-2 (Continued)

Citation (authors, year, title of article, journal, volume, issue, pages):		
Aims, research questions or hypotheses:		
Type:	Quantitative	Mixed methods
Study site:		
Sample:	Size:	Sampling plan:
	Demographics:	
Variables and instruments	Dependent:	
	Independent (including intervention):	
	Potential confounding:	

Figure 4-3 Literature review worksheet for quantitative research in a table.

Design	Experimental			Nonexperimental				
	Randomized controlled trial			Cohort study				
	Experiment			Case control study				
	Quasi-experimental			Descriptive comparative study				
				Descriptive correlation study				
				Descriptive, exploratory study				
Results:								
Recommendations:								

Figure 4-3 (*Continued*)

Strengths: Internal validity:	External validity
Limitations: Internal validity:	External validity

ANALYSIS

Clinical significance:	
Credibility of results:	
Intervention applicable to my setting:	
Acceptability of benefit vs. risk:	
Acceptability of costs:	

Figure 4-3 (*Continued*)

Citation (authors, year, title of article, journal, volume, issue, pages):			
Purpose, aims, or research questions:			
Research tradition:			
Content analysis ———	Grounded theory ———	Ethnography ———	Mixed methods ———	Other
Study site:			
Sample:			
Size: ———	Sampling plan: ———	Demographics:	
Phenomenon of interest			
Results:			
Recommendations:			

Figure 4-4 Literature review worksheet for qualitative research studies.

Appraisal questions:		
Did researcher report preconceptions or biases?		
Was the research tradition appropriate for the purpose of the study?		
If there was a theoretical framework, was it appropriate for the research tradition?		
Were the data collection procedures appropriate for the research tradition?		
Were included informants appropriate for the purpose of the study?		
Did data collection continue until redundancy or data saturation reached?		
Is analysis described with sufficient detail that another researcher could replicate the study?		
Is the description of results appropriate for the research tradition?		

Figure 4-4 (*Continued*)

Does discussion include linkages of results to existing knowledge?							
Trustworthiness							
Credibility:							
Dependability:							
Confirmability							
Transferability							
ANALYSIS							
Clinical significance:							
Intervention applicable to my setting:							
Acceptability of benefit vs. risk:							
Acceptability of costs:							

Figure 4-4 (*Continued*)

Introduction and Literature Review Sections
1. What is the problem statement for the study?
2. What was the purpose?
3. What was the hypothesis?
4. What were the research questions?
5. What concepts are explored? Is there an independent variable? A dependent variable?
6. Was the need for the study adequately justified? (Author identified gaps in existing literature.) What was the justification?

Methodology Section
1. What was the dependent variable? Independent variable? Other measured variables?
2. How were the variables measured?
3. Did the instrument(s) have good psychometric properties (validity; reliability)?
4. Who is the target population to be studied? Was the most informative population sampled?
5. Was the sample representative of the target population?
6. What was the sampling plan? Did it minimize selection bias while maximizing representativeness?
7. Did the author justify sample size?
8. How did the researcher control extraneous variables?
9. Were the statistical analyses appropriate for the level of data?
10. Was the analysis adequate to answer the research questions?

Results and Discussion Sections
1. Were the research questions answered in the results section?
2. What implications for practice are described by the researchers?
3. Were these implications supported by this study's findings?
4. Can you think of additional implications?
5. What future research did the researchers suggest?
6. Can you suggest additional research built upon this study's findings?

Other
What are the strengths of the study?
What are the major limitations of the study?
What design improvements could you suggest?

Figure 4-5   Checklist for collecting data about quantitative studies.

Methodology Checklist 1: Systematic Reviews and Meta-analyses	
Title of practice change project:	Team name:
PICO Question:	C:
P:	O:
I:	
Checklist completed by:	
Section 1: Internal validity	

In a well-conducted systematic review		In this study this criterion is	
1.1	The study addresses an appropriate and clearly focused question.	Well-covered	Not addressed
		Adequately addressed	Not reported
		Poorly addressed	Not applicable
1.2	A description of the methodology used is included.	Well-covered	Not addressed
		Adequately addressed	Not reported
		Poorly addressed	Not applicable
1.3	The literature search is sufficiently rigorous to identify all the relevant studies.	Well-covered	Not addressed
		Adequately addressed	Not reported
		Poorly addressed	Not applicable
1.4	Study quality is assessed and taken into account.	Well-covered	Not addressed
		Adequately addressed	Not reported
		Poorly addressed	Not applicable

Figure 4-6   Checklist for appraising systematic reviews.

1.5	There are enough similarities between the studies selected to make combining them reasonable.	Well-covered	Not addressed
		Adequately addressed	Not reported
		Poorly addressed	Not applicable

Section 2: Overall assessment of the study

| 2.1 | **How well was the study done to minimize bias?** **Code ++, +, or −** | |
| 2.2 | If coded as +, or − what is the likely direction in which bias might affect the study results? | |

Section 3: Description of the study (Please print answers clearly)

3.1	What types of study are included in the review? *(Highlight all that apply)*	RCT CCT Cohort
		Case-control Other
3.2	How does this review help to answer your key question? *Summarize the main conclusions of the review and how it relates to the relevant key question. Comment on any particular strengths or weaknesses of the review as a source of evidence for a guideline produced for the NHS in Scotland.*	

Adapted with permission by the Scottish Intercollegiate Guidelines Network (SIGN) from SIGN Methodology Checklist 1

Figure 4-6   (*Continued*)

There are critical appraisal tools available online for appraising the internal validity of CPGs. A recently developed tool is entitled the AGREE instrument. AGREE is the abbreviation for Appraisal of Guidelines Research and Evaluation. It was developed by an international collaboration of researchers and policy makers from European countries and the United States. The stimulus for this collaboration was concern about the inconsistent quality and rigor of some CPGs. The AGREE collaboration began in 1998 with the aim of improving the quality of CPGs by developing a shared framework for their development, reporting, and assessment.[65,66] The project to develop the instrument was coordinated by the Department of Public Health Sciences at St. George's Hospital Medical School in London. In 2006, the copyright and responsibility for the AGREE instrument was transferred to the AGREE Research Trust. The internal validity criteria for CPGs that make up the AGREE instrument are displayed in Figure 4-7. The AGREE instrument and its training manual can be obtained free from http://www.agreetrust.org/.

Another site for accessing a tool for appraising CPGs is the Evidence-Based Medicine Toolkit, http://www.ebm.med.ualberta.ca/.

The Centre for Evidence-Based Medicine has free downloadable software called CATmaker that helps the user to generate critical appraisal topics (CATs) that equate to the completed appraisal of the research report about the *effectiveness of an intervention*. CATmaker can be downloaded from http://www.cebm.net/index.aspx?o=1157. CATmaker performs the following functions:

- Prompts for the research question for the review, search strategy, and key information about the study found.
- Provides online critical appraisal guides for assessing the validity and usefulness of the study.
- Automates the calculation of clinically useful measures.
- Helps formulate clinical "bottom lines" based on all the information.
- Creates one-page summaries (CATs) that are easy to store, print, retrieve, and share (as both text and HTML files).

SCOPE AND PURPOSE
1. The overall objective(s) of the guideline is (are) specifically described.
2. The clinical question(s) covered by the guideline is (are) specifically described.
3. The patients to whom the guideline is meant to apply are specifically described.

STAKEHOLDER INVOLVEMENT
4. The guideline development group includes individuals from all the relevant professional groups.
5. The patients' views and preferences have been sought.
6. The target users of the guideline are clearly defined.
7. The guideline has been piloted among target users.

RIGOUR OF DEVELOPMENT
8. Systematic methods were used to search for evidence.
9. The criteria for selecting the evidence are clearly described.
10. The methods used for formulating the recommendations are clearly described.
11. The health benefits, side effects, and risks have been considered in formulating the recommendations.
12. There is an explicit link between the recommendations and the supporting evidence.
13. The guideline has been externally reviewed by experts prior to its publication.
14. A procedure for updating the guideline is provided.
15. The recommendations are specific and unambiguous.
16. The different options for management of the condition are clearly presented.
17. Key recommendations are easily identifiable.
18. The guideline is supported with tools for application.
19. The potential organizational barriers in applying the recommendations have been discussed.
20. The potential cost implications of applying the recommendations have been considered.
21. The guideline presents key review criteria for monitoring and/or audit purposes.
22. The guideline is editorially independent from the funding body.
23. Conflicts of interest of guideline development members have been recorded.

*Uses a 4-point response scale with 1 = strongly disagree and 4 = strongly agree

Figure 4-7   AGREE instrument* criteria for internal validity of a CPG. Used with permission from AGREE Collaboration. (2007). Appraisal of Guidelines for Research & Evaluation. Retrieved July 20, 2007, from http://www.agreecollaboration.org/intro/.

• Reminds when to update each CAT.
• Helps to teach others how to practice EBP.

The EBP team must complete data collection about the included research articles before using CATmaker. Use of this software is an advanced skill. Therefore, depending on the previous research experience, computer skills, interest of team members, and time, the team may wish to defer considering the use of CATmaker until after it has successfully completed at least one EBP project.

Choose or Design an Evidence Table Template for Displaying Data about Research Evidence

The EBP team should plan on inputting data from the critical appraisal tools into an evidence table after data about each research article have been collected. Organizing the key information into an evidence table will make it easier for the team to analyze all the research evidence and write the synthesis. An example of an evidence table template for quantitative research appears in Figure 4-8, and an example of an evidence table template for qualitative research appears in Figure 4-9.

Systematic reviews by the Cochrane Collaboration typically include a separate table displaying the characteristics of included studies and the characteristics of excluded studies. They may include additional tables, such as a summary of adverse outcomes or the quality of the included studies. The characteristics of included studies consist of

• Methods
• Participants, site, and country
• Interventions
• Outcomes
• Notes

The table for the characteristics of excluded studies consists of a brief explanation of why the study failed to meet the inclusion criteria.

Author, Date	Aims, Research Questions, or Hypotheses	Methodology: Design, Site, Sample	Intervention	Variables and Instruments	Results	Strengths and Limitations

Figure 4-8   Evidence table template for quantitative research.

Citation	Purpose, Aims, or Research Questions	Methodology: Design, Site, Sample	Phenomenon of Interest	Results	Strengths and Limitations

Figure 4-9 Evidence table template for qualitative research.

Synthesis Worksheet

A. Write clear, concise statements about the findings that are supported by the evidence and identify the supportive evidence.

1.

2.

3.

B. Write statements regarding whether the body of evidence is homogeneous (consistent) or heterogeneous (inconsistent).

1.

2.

3.

C. If the body of evidence is heterogeneous (inconsistent), write explicit statements regarding plausible explanations for the inconsistencies. (Tip: they are usually due to how well the design of a study is controlled for threats to internal validity or a sample size too small to have enough power to detect an intervention's effect or a difference. You would usually have more confidence in studies designed to control for threats to interval validity with adequate sample sizes than other studies.)

1.

2.

3.

D. Write clear, explicit statements about the remaining gaps in the knowledge base.

1.

2.

3.

E. Based on your critical analysis of the evidence, write conclusions regarding the adequacy of the evidence to support a practice change.

1.

2.

3.

Figure 4-10 Synthesis worksheet template.

Synthesis

A synthesis is a summary of the current state of knowledge about the topic that was the focus of the literature review. The EBP team will write the synthesis after critically analyzing the evidence summarized in the evidence tables and the summaries of critical appraisal of systematic reviews and CPGs, if such are located. The team can prepare for the activity of writing a synthesis by critically examining the syntheses in systematic reviews or by critically examining the syntheses that appear before the methods section in research reports. There are educational handouts on various aspects of writing on many university writing center web sites that can be located by an Internet browser search. However, university students are the target audience for these handouts, and so they may not be an efficient resource for direct-care nurses. A synthesis worksheet template that may help EBP team members write a synthesis is in Figure 4-10.

CONDUCT THE SEARCH

Once the EBP team has finished its planning for conducting its systematic review on the project topic, it is ready to begin conducting the search. This can be an adventure for the novice searcher because the electronic databases have different search tools. Some databases' search tools are quite simple but have limited options for designing highly selective searches. Others, like PubMed, have many options for designing highly selective searches. Some databases provide only the citation of the reference and an abstract, whereas others have links to electronic copies of the full text of the reference.

Learning to Search Using Electronic Databases

Resources for learning how to use various databases will depend largely upon the team's work setting. Health-care organizations that are affiliated with a university or that have a library may have educational offerings about how to use databases available in that organization, such as live classes, handouts, archived webcasts, or online tutorials. Team members should contact a librarian at their local health science library to inquire about the availability of educational materials. Many proprietary databases are available from more than one vendor, and the search features can vary by vendor. They can also vary by the version of the database because enhancements are made periodically. The educational materials should be for the current version of the database. There are short tutorials for using PubMed online (Appendix J).

Tips for Searching for the Evidence

The goal is to find the literature relevant to the EBP project. Following these tips helps make the most efficient use of time in the task of searching:

• Keep a log (see Figure 4-11)

— Mark which keywords have been searched for in each available, relevant database.

— Write in how many reference "hits" there were for each combination of keywords.

— Make decisions about limiting or expanding the search based on the number of hits and their relevance to the project.

• When relevant hits are obtained, print them, if that option is available. Also, it is helpful to save the citation, abstract, or PDF, if available, to a disk or your hard drive.

— By saving the file, the team can

▪ create a "virtual" library by saving the PDF in a folder labeled with the name of the project and

▪ generate an electronic reference list without handwriting or typing, with the accompanying risk of making errors.

— For instance, PubMed provides the option to "send" a citation or a group of selected citations to a text file, which the team members can use to generate a list of citations of references they want to retrieve.

Key search words

A. Patient or problem of interest _____

B. Main intervention _____

C. Comparison intervention _____

D. Primary outcome of interest _____

E. Secondary outcomes of interest _____

Key Words & Combinations	National Guidelines Clearinghouse	Cochrane Library	Full-Text Databases Years Searched:	PubMed Years Searched:	CINAHL Years Searched:

Figure 4-11   Literature search log.

- ■ To also download the abstract, the "display" format must be switched from "summary" to "Medline."
- Search for CPGs and systematic reviews first.
- Then, search PubMed.
- Next, separately search CINAHL and all the relevant, available databases.
- When searching PubMed, CINAHL, and the full-text databases, search separately for review articles and research articles.
- Search specialty databases (PsycINFO, Social Sciences Abstracts, and other such resources) if they are appropriate for your topic.
- Examine the titles and abstracts of the obtained hits, choosing the ones for which you wish to obtain a copy.
  - — Make a list to use in retrieving and organizing evidence documents.

Using a search log can help the EBP team avoid repeating searches of keywords and databases. That can easily happen as variations in the combinations of keywords are made for thoroughness and to help limit excessive numbers of hits. An example of how to use the log appears in Figure 4-12. This search log uses the keywords from the PICO question for the fabricated CHF EBP project. The first column contains the keywords as they were actually entered. The databases were searched from left to right and included all relevant databases accessible to the author. A smaller number of keywords results in large quantities of hits that would be difficult to read through. Incrementally adding more keywords resulted in smaller numbers of hits and a higher percentage of hits that were relevant to the PICO question. Adding limits, such as how many years to search, field location (title, abstract, and so on) for the keyword, and type of publication (research, review, and so on), helped narrow some searches to more relevant articles. Following are examples of searches.

Key search words:

A. Patient or problem of interest: Chronic heart failure patients

B. Main intervention: Long-term management by a nurse practitioner

C. Comparison intervention: Patient teaching of self-care by a staff nurse

D. Primary outcome of interest: Unplanned readmission in less that 30 days due to inadequate self-care

E. Secondary outcomes of interest: _____

Key Words & Combinations	National Guidelines Clearinghouse	Cochrane Library	Full-Text Databases Years searched: 10 years	PubMed Years searched: 10 years	CINAHL Years searched: 10 years
- Chronic heart failure - Education	20 hits, 3 highly relevant	118 hits, narrowed with more key words	55 hits, to narrow, limited to chronic heart failure appearing in title; 20 hits with 5 relevant	385 hits, to narrow search, added limits to RCTs and comparative studies and limited to 10 years back; 18 of 63 hits were relevant	82 hits, narrowed with more key words
- Chronic heart failure in title		16, not relevant	1002 hits, narrowed with more key words	1221 hits, narrowed with more key words	671 hits, narrowed with more key words
- Chronic heart failure - Nurse practitioner - Readmission		2 hits, not on target	0 hits	1 hit, relevant	0 hits
- Chronic heart failure - Teaching		0 hits	16 hits, not relevant	20 hits, 5 relevant	11 hits, 5 relevant
- Chronic heart failure - Education	20 hits, 3 highly relevant	118 hits, narrowed with more key words	55 hits, narrowed with more key words	385 hits, to narrow search, added limits to RCTs and comparative studies and limited to 10 years back; 18 of 63 hits were relevant	82 hits, narrowed with more key words

Figure 4-12   Example of a completed literature search log.

- Chronic heart failure - Readmission		1 hit, not relevant	25 hits, 9 relevant	49 hits, narrowed with more key words	18 hits, 12 relevant
- Chronic heart failure - Education - Nurse		9 hits, relevant	5 hits, 3 relevant	10 hit, 6 relevant	14, 9 relevant
- Heart failure - Education - Nurse - Readmission		1 hit, not relevant because studies with educational interventions were omitted	8 hits, 5 relevant	13 hits, 10 relevant	22 this, 18 relevant
- Chronic heart failure - nurse practitioner - Education			1 hit, not relevant	1 hit, not relevant	0 hits

Figure 4-12   (*Continued*)

Examples of Searching for Evidence

Examples of searches of two publicly available electronic databases, the National Guideline Clearinghouse and PubMed, appear below. The examples are for the fabricated case on CHF introduced in Step 1, using the PICO question for CHF (Case 3-2.E):

In CHF patients with unplanned readmission in less than 30 days due to inadequate self-care, will long-term management by a nurse practitioner be more effective than patient teaching of self-care by a staff nurse in reducing the number of unplanned readmissions within 30 days of discharge by 10 percent?

The ultimate desired outcome for the fabricated CHF EBP project was to reduce unplanned readmissions to the hospital less than 30 days after discharge. Inclusion criteria were

- CHF patients
- Long-term management by a nurse practitioner
- Patient teaching of self-care by a direct-care nurse
- The number of unplanned readmissions within 30 days of discharge

- Published in the last 10 years
- RCTs and comparative research studies
  — Limit to RCTs if there is a large number of RCT hits
- No limits on geographic location
- Type of health-care setting limited to acute-care settings, patients' home, and long-term care facilities

 CASE 4-2 *Searching for a Clinical Practice Guideline in the National Guidelines Clearinghouse*

- Search words "chronic heart failure AND education."
  — Obtained 20 hits.
  — After reviewing titles and scanning documents, two were relevant for the fabricated CHF project.[67,68]
- Both CPGs identified information that needed to be taught to the patient for self-care after discharge.

 CASE 4-3 *Searching for Systematic Reviews in PubMed*

- Search words "chronic heart failure AND education AND readmission AND nurse practitioner" with limits of 10 years and publication type as meta-analysis and review.
  — 0 hits
- Search words "chronic heart failure AND education AND *hospitalization* AND nurse" with limits of 10 years and publication type as meta-analysis and review.
  — 2 hits, both somewhat relevant
- Search words "chronic heart failure AND education AND *hospitalization* AND *self-care*" with limits of 10 years and publication type as meta-analysis and review.
  — 9 hits, 5 relevant

 CASE 4-4 *Searching for Research in PubMed*

- Search for "chronic heart failure AND education."
  — Obtained 385 hits
- To narrow the hits, add limits of RCTs and comparative studies published in the past 10 years.

— Obtained 63 hits.

— After examining the titles and abstracts, 18 of 63 looked potentially relevant.

 CASE 4-5 *Searching for Expert Committee Reports on Chronic Heart Failure in PubMed*

* Search words "expert committee reports AND chronic heart failure."
  — 1 hit
* Search words "consensus statements AND chronic heart failure."
  — 0 hits
* Type of publication limited to "consensus development conference" and "consensus development conference, NIH" and search words "heart failure."
  — 10 hits[69–78]

Once the EBP team members have located and obtained the best evidence relevant to the project topic, they move on to Step 3 to critically appraise the evidence and to weigh the strength of the evidence.

REFERENCES

1. Institute of Medicine. *Clinical Practice Guidelines: Directions for a New Program*. Washington, DC: National Academy Press; 1990.
2. McCormick KA, Fleming B. Clinical practice guidelines. The Agency for Health Care Policy and Research fosters the development of evidence-based guidelines. *Health Prog.* 1992;73(10): 30–34.
3. Klassen TP, Jadad AR, Moher D. Guides for reading and interpreting systematic reviews: I. Getting started. *Arch Pediatr Adolesc Med.* Jul 1998;152(7):700–704.
4. Greenhalgh T. Education and debate. How to read a paper: Papers that summarise other papers (systematic reviews and meta-analyses) . . . ninth in a series of 10 articles. *BMJ: British Medical Journal.* 1997;315(7109):672–675.

5. The Cochrane Collaboration. The Cochrane Collaboration Home Page. http://www.cochrane.org/index.htm. Accessed June 20, 2007.

6. The Campbell Collaboration. C2 Home Page. http://www.campbellcollaboration.org/index.asp. Accessed June 20, 2007.

7. Welcome to Evidence-Base On Call database. Top CATs. http://www.eboncall.org/content.jsp.htm. Accessed July 6, 2007.

8. Booth S, Wade R, Johnson M, et al. The use of oxygen in the palliation of breathlessness. A report of the expert working group of the Scientific Committee of the Association of Palliative Medicine. *Respir Med.* Jan 2004;98(1):66–77.

9. Harris RP, Helfand M, Woolf SH, et al. Current methods of the US Preventive Services Task Force: A review of the process. *Am J Prev Med.* Apr 2001;20(3 Suppl):21–35.

10. Polit DF, Beck CT. *Nursing Research: Generating and Assessing Evidence for Nursing Practice.* 8th ed. Philadelphia, PA: J. B. Lippincott; 2008.

11. BMJ Clinical Evidence. Glossary. http://www.clinicalevidence.com/ceweb/resources/glossary.jsp#C. Accessed July 5, 2007.

12. Borbasi S, Jackson D, Langford R. *Navigating the Maze of Nursing Research: An Interactive Learning Adventure.* Sydney: Mosby; 2004.

13. Oermann MH, Nordstrom CK, Wilmes NA, et al. Information sources for developing the nursing literature. *Int J Nurs Stud.* Dec 2 2006;doi:10.1016/j.ijnurstu.2006.10.005.

14. Hallal JC. Introduction to the research process: A primer for the practicing nurse. *J Hosp Palliat Nurs.* 1999;1(3):108–115.

15. Frame K, Kelly L. Reading nursing research: Easy as ABCD. *J Sch Nurs.* Dec 2003;19(6):326–329.

16. Fosbinder D, Loveridge C. How to critique a research study. *Adv Pract Nurs Q.* Winter 1996;2(3):68–71.

17. Ryan-Wenger NM. Guidelines for critique of a research report. *Heart Lung.* Jul-Aug 1992;21(4):394–401.

18. Miller B. The literature review. In: LoBiondo-Wood G, Haber J, eds. *Nursing Research: Methods, Critical Appraisal, and Utilization.* 3rd ed. St. Louis: Mosby; 1994: 109–141.

19. Evans JC, Shreve WS. The ASK Model: A bare bones approach to the critique of nursing research for use in practice. *J Trauma Nurs*. 2000;7(4):83–91.
20. Rasmussen L, O'Conner M, Shinkle S, Thomas MK. The basic research review checklist. *J Contin Educ Nurs*. 2000;31(1):13–17.
21. Pieper B. Basics of critiquing a research article. *J ET Nurs*. 1993;20:245–250.
22. Giuffre M. Reading research critically: Statistical significance. *J Post Anesth Nurs*. Dec 1994;9(6):371–374.
23. Giuffre M. Reading research critically: Threats to internal validity. *J Post Anesth Nurs*. Oct 1994;9(5):303–307.
24. Giuffre M. Reading research critically: The review of the literature. *J Post Anesth Nurs*. Aug 1994;9(4):240–243.
25. Giuffre M. Reading research critically: Results—bivariate regression analysis. *J Post Anesth Nurs*. Dec 1995;10(6):340–344.
26. Giuffre M. Reading research critically: Results using correlation coefficients. *J Post Anesth Nurs*. Aug 1995;10(4):220–224.
27. Giuffre M. Reading research critically: Results—Part 1. *J Post Anesth Nurs*. Jun 1995;10(3):166–171.
28. Giuffre M. Reading research critically: Assessing the validity and reliability of research instrumentation—Part 2. *J Post Anesth Nurs*. Apr 1995;10(2):107–112.
29. Giuffre M. Reading research critically: Assessing the validity and reliability of research instrumentation—Part 1. *J Post Anesth Nurs*. Feb 1995;10(1):33–37.
30. Giuffre M. Reading research critically: The discussion section. *J Perianesth Nurs*. Dec 1996;11(6):417–420.
31. Giuffre M. Reading research critically: Results—group data. *J Perianesth Nurs*. Oct 1996;11(5):344–348.
32. Giuffre M. Reading research critically: Results: Multiple regression analysis. *J Post Anesth Nurs*. Feb 1996;11(1):32–34.
33. Giuffre M. Reading research critically: Results—group data II. *J Perianesth Nurs*. Apr 1997;12(2):105–108.
34. Speziale HSC, Rinaldi D. *Qualitative Research in Nursing: Advancing the Humanistic Imperative*. 3rd ed. Philadelphia, PA: Lippincott Williams & Wilkins; 2003.

35. Guba EG. Criteria for assessing the trustworthiness of naturalistic inquiries. *Educational Communication and Technology Journal*. 1981;29:75–91.

36. Shenton AK. Strategies for ensuring trustworthiness in qualitative research projects. *Education for Information*. 2004;22(2): 63–75.

37. Greenhalgh T, Taylor R. Papers that go beyond numbers (qualitative research). *BMJ*. Sep 20 1997;315(7110):740–743.

38. Farley A, McLafferty E. An introduction to qualitative research concepts for nurses. *Prof Nurse*. Nov 2003;19(3):159–163.

39. Cote L, Turgeon J. Appraising qualitative research articles in medicine and medical education. *Med Teach*. Jan 2005;27(1): 71–75.

40. Lee P. Understanding some naturalistic research methodologies. *Paediatr Nurs*. Apr 2006;18(3):44–46.

41. Lee P. Understanding and critiquing qualitative research papers. *Nurs Times*. Jul 18–24 2006;102(29):30–32.

42. Thompson CB, Walker BL. Basics of research (Part 12): Qualitative research. *Air Med J*. Apr–Jun 1998;17(2): 65–70.

43. Barbour RS. The role of qualitative research in broadening the "evidence base" for clinical practice. *J Eval Clin Pract*. May 2000;6(2):155–163.

44. Greenhalgh T. Integrating qualitative research into evidence based practice. *Endocrinol Metab Clin North Am*. Sep 2002; 31(3):583–601, ix.

45. Ailinger RL. Contributions of qualitative research to evidence-based practice in nursing. *Revista Latino-Americana de Enfermagem*. May-Jun 2003;11(3):275–279.

46. Sandelowski M. Using qualitative research. *Qual Health Res*. Dec 2004;14(10):1366–1386.

47. Tripp-Reimer T, Doebbeling B. Qualitative perspectives in translational research. *Worldviews Evid Based Nurs*. 2004; 1 (Suppl 1):S65–S72.

48. Grypdonck MH. Qualitative health research in the era of evidence-based practice. *Qual Health Res*. Dec 2006;16(10): 1371–1385.

49. Sandelowski M, Trimble F, Woodard EK, Barroso J. From synthesis to script: Transforming qualitative research findings for use in practice. *Qual Health Res.* Dec 2006;16(10):1350–1370.

50. Corrrigan M, Cupples ME, Smith SM, et al. The contribution of qualitative research in designing a complex intervention for secondary prevention of coronary heart disease in two different healthcare systems. *BMC Health Serv Res.* 2006;6:90.

51. Morse JM, Penrod J, Hupcey JE. Qualitative outcome analysis: Evaluating nursing interventions for complex clinical phenomena. *J Nurs Scholarsh.* 2000;32(2):125–130.

52. Dickson R. Systematic Reviews. In: Hamer S, Collinson G, eds. *Achieving Evidence-Based Practice: A Handbook for Practitioners.* Edinburgh, Scotland: Elsevier; 2005:43–62.

53. Ganong LH. Integrative reviews of nursing research. *Res Nurs Health.* Feb 1987;10(1):1–11.

54. Cooper HM. *Synthesizing Research: A Guide for Literature Reviews.* Thousand Oaks, CA: Sage Publications; 1998.

55. Joanna Briggs Institute for Evidence Based Nursing and Midwifery. Changing practice: Appraising systematic reviews. *Changing Practice: Evidence Based Practice Information Sheets for Health Professionals.* 2000; http://www.joannabriggs.edu.au/ about/ home.php. Accessed May 20, 2007.

56. Jadad AR, Moher D, Klassen TP. Guides for reading and interpreting systematic reviews: II. How did the authors find the studies and assess their quality? *Arch Pediatr Adolesc Med.* 1998;152(8):812–817.

57. Moher D, Jadad AR, Klassen TP. Guides for reading and interpreting systematic reviews: III. How did the authors synthesize the data and make their conclusions? *Arch Pediatr Adolesc Med.* Sep 1998;152(9):915–920.

58. Oxman AD, Guyatt GH. The science of reviewing research. *Ann N Y Acad Sci.* 1993;703:125.

59. Centre for Evidence-Based Medicine. EBP Tools. http://www.cebm.net/index.aspx?o=1039. Accessed July 3, 2007.

60. Higgins J, Green S, eds. Cochrane Handbook for Systematic Reviews of Interventions 4.2.6. September 2006; http://www.cochrane.org/resources/handbook/. Accessed June 23, 2007.

61. Hill A, Spittlehouse C. What is critical appraisal? *Evid Based Med*. 2001;3(2):1–8.

62. Cesario S, Morin K, Santa-Donato A. Evaluating the level of evidence of qualitative research. *J Obstet Gynecol Neonatal Nurs*. Nov–Dec 2002;31(6):708–714.

63. Duffy ME. A research appraisal checklist for evaluating nursing research reports. *Nurs Health Care*. 1985;6: 539–547.

64. Rosswurm MA, Larrabee JH. A model for change to evidence-based practice. *Image J Nurs Sch*. 1999;31(4):317–322.

65. AGREE Collaboration. Appraisal of Guidelines for Research & Evaluation. http://www.agreecollaboration.org/intro/. Accessed July 20, 2007.

66. Burgers JS, Grol R, Klazinga NS, et al. Towards evidence-based clinical practice: An international survey of 18 clinical guideline programs. *Int J Qual Health Care*. Feb 2003;15(1): 31–45.

67. Scottish Intercollegiate Guidelines Network (SIGN). Management of chronic heart failure: A national clinical guideline. February 2007; available through the National Guidelines Clearinghouse, http://www.guideline.gov/. Accessed July 19, 2007.

68. Swedberg K, Cleland J, Dargie H, et al. Guidelines for the diagnosis and treatment of chronic heart failure. 2005; available through the National Guidelines Clearinghouse, http://www.guideline.gov/. Accessed July 19, 2007.

69. Arnold JM, Howlett JG, Dorian P, et al. Canadian Cardiovascular Society Consensus Conference recommendations on heart failure update 2007: Prevention, management during intercurrent illness or acute decompensation, and use of biomarkers. *Can J Cardiol*. Jan 2007;23(1):21–45.

70. Hooper WC, Catravas JD, Heistad DD, et al. Vascular endothelium summary statement I: Health promotion and chronic disease prevention. *Vascul Pharmacol*. May 2007; 46(5):315–317.

71. Ly J, Chan CT. Impact of augmenting dialysis frequency and duration on cardiovascular function. *Asaio J*. Nov-Dec 2006;52(6):e11–e14.

72. Quinones MA, Zile MR, Massie BM, Kass DA. Chronic heart failure: A report from the Dartmouth Diastole Discourses. *Congest Heart Fail*. May-Jun 2006;12(3):162–165.

73. Anker SD, John M, Pedersen PU, et al. ESPEN Guidelines on Enteral Nutrition: Cardiology and pulmonology. *Clin Nutr.* Apr 2006;25(2):311–318.

74. Cavill I, Auerbach M, Bailie GR, et al. Iron and the anaemia of chronic disease: A review and strategic recommendations. *Curr Med Res Opin*. Apr 2006;22(4):731–737.

75. Clark WR, Paganini E, Weinstein D, et al. Extracorporeal ultrafiltration for acute exacerbations of chronic heart failure: Report from the Acute Dialysis Quality Initiative. *Int J Artif Organs*. May 2005;28(5):466–476.

76. Wyrwich KW, Spertus JA, Kroenke K, et al. Clinically important differences in health status for patients with heart disease: An expert consensus panel report. *Am Heart J.* Apr 2004; 147(4):615–622.

77. Consensus recommendations for the management of chronic heart failure. On behalf of the membership of the advisory council to improve outcomes nationwide in heart failure. *Am J Cardiol*. Jan 21 1999;83(2A):1A–38A.

78. Burkart F, Erdmann E, Hanrath P, et al. [Consensus conference "Therapy of chronic heart insufficiency" inaugurated by the Munich Collegium for Therapy Research e.V. together with the German Society for Cardiovascular Research]. *Z Kardiol*. Mar 1993;82(3):200–210.

79. West Virginia University Libraries. Databases: Health Sciences & Medicine. http://www.libraries.wvu.edu/databases/cgi-bin/databases.pl?type=32. Accessed June 22, 2007.

80. School of Health and Related Research (ScHARR). ScHARR Guides. http://www.shef.ac.uk/scharr/ir/units/. Accessed July 4, 2007.

81. University of Minnesota. Evidence-based health care project. http://evidence.ahc.umn.edu/. Accessed July 6, 2007.

82. University of Minnesota. Evidence-based nursing. http://evidence.ahc.umn.edu/ebn.htm. Accessed July 5, 2007.

83. Scottish Intercollegiate Guidelines Network. Critical appraisal: Notes and checklists. http://www.sign.ac.uk/ methodology/ checklists.html. Accessed July 3, 2007.

84. Brown SJ. *Knowledge for Health Care Practice: A Guide to Using Research Evidence*. Philadelphia, PA: W. B. Saunders; 1999.

85. Critical Appraisal Skills Programme and Evidence-Based Practice (CASP). Critical Appraisal Tools. http:// www.phru.nhs.uk/casp/ critical_appraisal_tools.htm#rct. Accessed July 2007.

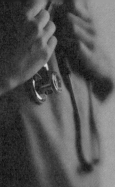

INTERNET SOURCES FOR CLINICAL PRACTICE GUIDELINES

- National Guideline Clearinghouse (NGC)
  —http://www.guidelines.gov/
- Centers for Disease Control and Prevention (CDC)
  —http://www.cdc.gov/
- Agency for Health Care Research and Quality
  —http://www.ahrq.gov/clinic/cpgonline.htm
- Health Canada
  —http://www.hc-sc.gc.ca/
- Canadian Task Force on Preventive Health Care
  —http://www.ctfphc.org/
- Scottish Intercollegiate Guidelines Network (SIGN)
  —http://www.sign.ac.uk/
- New Zealand Guidelines Group
  —www.nzgg.org.nz
- Institute for Clinical Systems Improvement (ICSI)
  —www.icsi.org
- European Society of Cardiology
  —http://www.escardio.org
- National Kidney Foundation
  —http://www.kidney.org/professionals/KDOQI/guidelines.cfm

- **Royal College of Obstetricians and Gynaecologists-**
  —http://www.rcog.org.uk
- **Infectious Diseases Society of America**
  —http://www.idsociety.org/pg/toc.htm
- **NHSHTA-click on "list of all HTA reports"**
  —http://www.hta.nhsweb.nhs.uk/

  Sites specific for nursing best practice guidelines include

- **Registered Nurses Association of Ontario—Best Practice Guidelines available for purchase**
  —http://www.rnao.org/bestpractices/index.asp
- **JBI ConNect by Joanna Briggs Institute for Evidence Based Nursing and Midwifery—subscription fee**
  —http://www.jbiconnect.org/index.php
- **University of Iowa Gerontological Nursing Interventions Research Center—guidelines available for purchase**
  —http://www.nursing.uiowa.edu/consumers_patients/evidence_based.htm
- **Association of Women's Health, Obstetric, and Neonatal Nurses (AWHONN) Standards and Guidelines—available for purchase**
  —http://www.awhonn.org/awhonn/
- **Emergency Nursing World**
  —http://www.enw.org/TOC.htm
- **American Association of periOperative Nurses—Practice Resources, available for purchase**
  —http://www.aorn.org/
- **McGill University Health Centre—Links to Guidelines**
  —http://muhc-ebn.mcgill.ca/index.html

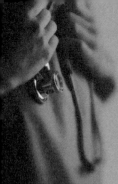

OTHER DATABASES FOR SYSTEMATIC REVIEWS

- **Health Services/Technology Assessment (HSTAT) home page**
  —http://hstat.nlm.nih.gov/
- **Clinical Evidence (subscription)**
  —www.clinicalevidence.com/uhf
- **Evidence-Based Practice Centers—Agency for Health Care Research and Quality**
  —http://www.ahrq.gov/clinic/epcquick.htm
- **Centre for Review and Dissemination**
  —http://www.york.ac.uk/inst/crd/
- **Bandolier—Abstracts of Systematic Reviews**
  —http://www.jr2.ox.ac.uk/bandolier/

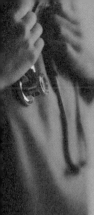

ONLINE BIBLIOGRAPHIC DATABASES WITH FREE ACCESS

- National Library of Medicine Gateway—http://gateway. nlm.nih.gov/gw/Cmd. This has information for health-care professional and consumers in a number of databases. For health-care professionals, they include

  —Medline/PubMed—journal citations and abstracts

  —NLM catalog—books, AVs, serials

  —BookShelf—full-text biomedical books

  —TOXLINE—toxicology citations

  —DART—developmental and reproductive toxicology

  —ClinicalTrials.gov

  —DIRLINE—Director of Health Organizations

  —Genetics Home Reference

  —Household Products Database

  —ITER—International Toxicology Estimates for Risk

  —GENE—TOX-Genetics Toxicology

  —CCRIS—Chemical Carcinogenesis Research Information System

- **PubMed (direct link)—http://www.ncbi.nlm.nih.gov/sites/ entrez**

    —A National Library of Medicine bibliographic database that indexes the medicine, nursing, dentistry, veterinary medicine and preclinical sciences literature in 4,600+ biomedical journals published in 70+ countries.

- **Cancer Literature in PubMed—http://www.cancer.gov/ search/cancer_literature/**

    —Links to search engines that are restricted to cancer literature

- **BioMed Central—http://www.biomedcentral.com/**

    —Publisher of 178 peer-reviewed open-access journals. The web site is searchable, and articles can be downloaded free.

- **AgeLine—http://www.aarp.org/research/ageline/**

    —A bibliographic database that abstracts 600 journal titles as well as books, chapters, research reports, and videos covering social gerontology and aging-related research.

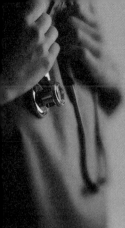

ONLINE BIBLIOGRAPHIC DATABASES ACCESSIBLE FOR A FEE

Because these databases are proprietary, access requires a username and password. Available proprietary databases include[79]

- **Academic Search Premiere**

  —A scholarly, multidisciplinary full-text database covering nearly all areas of academic study and containing full text for 4,650 periodicals.

  —In addition to the full text, this database offers indexing and abstracts for more than 8,200 journals.

- **HealthSource Nursing/Academic Edition**

  —Provides nearly 600 scholarly full-text journals, including nearly 450 peer-reviewed journals focusing on many medical disciplines.

  —Also provides abstracts and indexing for nearly 850 journals.

- **MDConsult**

  —Provides electronic access to 40 respected medical reference books, over 50 medical journals and clinics, MEDLINE, comprehensive drug information, more than 1,000 CPGs and over 3,500 customizable patient education handouts that patients can take home after an office visit or hospital stay.

—Online CME MD Consult provides online continuing medical education (CME).

- **CINAHL (Cumulative Index of Nursing and Allied Health Literature) with Full Text**

    —The world's most comprehensive source of full text for nursing and allied health journals, providing 600,000+ full-text articles from 550+ journals.

- **The Cochrane Library**

    —Includes the Cochrane Central Register of Controlled Trials.

- **PsycINFO**

    —Contains nearly two million citations and summaries of journal articles, book chapters, books, and dissertations, all in the field of psychology

- **EMBASE**

    —A European bibliographic database that indexes pharmacological and biomedical literature in 7,000+ journals from over 70 countries.

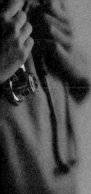

CRITICAL APPRAISAL TOPIC WEB SITES

- **University of North Carolina-CATs**
  —http://www.med.unc.edu/medicine/edursrc/welcome
- **Scottish Intensive Care—CATs**
  —http://www.sicsebm.org.uk/cat_collection.htm
- **University of Michigan**
  —http://www.med.umich.edu/pediatrics/ebm/topics/cards.htm
- **Evidence-Based On Call**
  —http://www.eboncall.org/content.jsp.htm
- **McMaster University Occupational Therapy Department**
  —http://www.srs-mcmaster.ca/Default.aspx?tabid=547

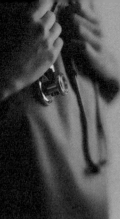

WEB SITES WITH NURSING POSITION STATEMENTS OR STANDARDS OF PRACTICE

- **American Nurses Association (ANA)**

    —http://nursingworld.org/

- **Association of Women's Health, Obstetric, and Neonatal Nurses (AWHONN) Standards and Guidelines—available for purchase**

    —http://www.awhonn.org/awhonn/

- **American Association of periOperative Nurses—Practice Resources, available for purchase**

    —http://www.aorn.org/

- **Links to other nursing organization web sites include**

    —ANA's Nursing Links (USA)—http://nursingworld.org/rnindex/snp.htm

    —Yahoo: Nursing Organizations (international)—http://dir.yahoo.com/health/nursing/organizations/

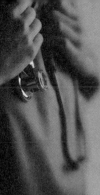

ONLINE RESEARCH EDUCATION RESOURCES

The School of Health and Related Research (ScHARR) of the University of Sheffield,[80] http://www.shef.ac.uk/scharr/ir/netting/, provides numerous resource links within eight web pages: library, searching, appraising, implementing, software, journals, databases, and organizations. On the library web page are links to electronic copies of educational articles about EBP. On this page, http://www.shef.ac.uk/scharr/ir/units/critapp/, is access to the following online education modules:

- Critical appraisal and using the literature
- Systematic reviews
- Getting research into practice

University of Minnesota,[81,82] http://evidence.ahc.umn.edu/ and http://evidence.ahc.umn.edu/ebn.htm, has educational modules about EBP and evidence-based nursing.

Evidence-Based Medicine, http://www.evidence-based-medicine.co.uk/; click on the "What is..." link to access educational materials about EBP, including "What is Critical Appraisal?"

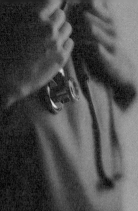

ONLINE EDUCATIONAL RESOURCES FOR QUALITATIVE RESEARCH

- **University of Sheffield, Netting the Evidence:**
  —http://www.shef.ac.uk/scharr/ir/units/
- **University of Kent:**
  —http://library.kent.ac.uk/library/info/subjectg/healthinfo/
  critapprais.shtml
- **Centre for Health Evidence**
  —http://www.cche.net/usersguides/qualitative.asp
- **The Qualitative Report, an online journal:**
  —http://www.nova.edu/ssss/QR/text.html

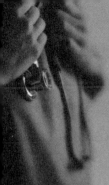

WEB SITES WITH CRITICAL APPRAISAL TOOLS

Systematic Reviews

Critical appraisal tools for appraising systematic reviews can be accessed online. Online resources include the following:

- The Scottish Intercollegiate Guideline Network has a checklist for appraising systematic reviews, explanatory notes about how to use it, and a copy available as a rtf that can be downloaded for typing in the critical appraisal.[83]

  —http://www.sign.ac.uk/guidelines/fulltext/50/checklist1.html

  A modified version of this checklist appears in Figure 4-7.

- Evidence-Based Medicine Toolkit has a collection of tools for appraising systematic reviews.

  —http://www.ebm.med.ualberta.ca/

- Joanna Briggs Institute for Evidence Based Nursing and Midwifery has a checklist for appraising systematic reviews with discussion about how to conduct the critical appraisal. http://www.joannabriggs.edu.au/about/home.php

  —Click on EBP Resources & Services, then

  —Click on Best Practice Information Sheet Database

  —Scroll to the sheet entitled "Changing Practice: Appraising Systematic Reviews" to download the PDF.

Quantitative Research Reports

Critical appraisal tools for appraising quantitative research reports can be accessed in the literature[19,84, pp 106–108] as well as online. Online resources include the following:

- Critical Appraisal Skills Programme and Evidence-Based Practice (CASP)[85] http://www.phru.nhs.uk/casp/critical_appraisal_tools.htm#rct has tools for appraising

    —RCTs

    —Qualitative research studies

    —Case control studies

    —Cohort studies

    —Economic evaluation studies

    —Diagnostic test studies

- The Scottish Intercollegiate Guideline Network has check-lists for the same types of evidence, as well as explanatory notes about how to use each tool.[83] http://www.sign.ac.uk/methodology/checklists.html

    —RCTs

    —Case control studies

    —Cohort studies

    —Economic evaluations studies

- Evidence-Based Medicine Toolkit, http://www.ebm.med.ualberta.ca/, has tools for appraising

    —RCTs

    —Economic evaluations studies

- McMaster University, Occupational Therapy Evidence-Based Practice Group http://www.srs-mcmaster.ca/Default.aspx?tabid=630 has tools and guidelines for appraising quantitative research studies.

Qualitative Research Reports

Critical appraisal tools for appraising qualitative research reports can be accessed in the literature[39,62] as well as online. Online resources include the following:

- University of Salford

  Critical appraisal tools:

  —http://www.fhsc.salford.ac.uk/hcprdu/tools/qualitative.htm

- McMaster University Occupational Therapy Evidence-Based Practice Group

  Critical appraisal guidelines and critical appraisal form

  —http://www.srs-mcmaster.ca/Default.aspx?tabid=630

- University of Southern California

  Health Science Evidence-Based Decision Making

  —http://www.usc.edu/hsc/ebnet/

  Making sense of the qualitative literature (a checklist)

  —http://www.usc.edu/hsc/ebnet/res/Making%20Sense%20of%20the%20QL%20Lit.pdf

- University of Connecticut

  Evaluation guidelines for qualitative research studies

  —www.isipar08.org/docs/Qualitative-Research-Criteria.doc

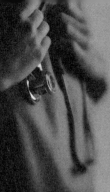

http://www.ncbi.nlm.nih.gov/sites/entrez

These include

- Search PubMed for an Author
- Searching PubMed by Author and Subject
- PubMed Simple Subject Search Example
- Search for a Journal
- Retrieving Citations from a Journal Issue

PubMed also has the option of registering for "My NCBI," which allows the user to save searches for later reference. There are a number of short tutorials about how to use My NCBI, including

- Getting Started with My NCBI
- How to register, sign in and out, change your password, and what to do if you've forgotten your password
- Saving Searches
- How to save a PubMed search, to run later or to have results sent to your e-mail account.
- How to save citations using My NCBI.
- E-mail Alerts for Articles from Your Favorite Journals
- How to create e-mail alerts for new articles from a set of journals.

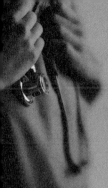

Chapter 5

STEP 3: CRITICALLY ANALYZE THE EVIDENCE

CRITIQUE AND WEIGH THE EVIDENCE

In this step, the evidence-based practice (EBP) team critically appraises the best evidence available that is relevant to the project's goal. Next, the team weighs the strength of the evidence, judging whether or not the evidence supports a practice change. If it does, the team considers whether or not the practice change supported by the evidence has acceptable feasibility, benefits, and risks.

Critiquing the Evidence

Having identified and obtained copies of the evidence, the team collects data about each clinical practice guideline, systematic review, and research report, using the tools selected while planning for conducting its systematic review. Team members should follow through with their plans to share the tasks of conducting the critical appraisals.

Clinical practice guidelines

If the team located a relevant clinical practice guideline (CPG), members should use the selected critical appraisal tool to appraise the CPG's internal validity. The AGREE instrument may seem challenging because it is 20 pages long and has 23 criteria for CPG internal validity. However, in addition to the critical appraisal form, there are pages that provide interpretations of each criterion, making the instrument less challenging to use than it first appears. There are examples of critical appraisals of CPGs using the AGREE instrument on this web site: http://www.agreecollaboration.org/1/agreeguide/.

 CASE 5-1 *Critical Appraisal of Two CPGs on Chronic Heart Failure Management*

The EBP team for the fabricated chronic heart failure (CHF) project had two relevant CPGs to critically appraise.[1,2] The team started with the one produced by the Scottish Intercollegiate Guidelines Network (SIGN), but when they were halfway through the 23 criteria, the team members became concerned because the guideline did not include some of the information pertaining to the criteria. For instance, it did not state the objective of the guideline or whether patients were included as stakeholders in the guideline development process. One team member browsed the SIGN web site, found a link to a description of the methodology followed in the development of all SIGN CPGs, and discovered that the process uses the AGREE instrument criteria. Thus, nurses using a SIGN CPG can have confidence that it has internal validity, even if they cannot highly rate some of the AGREE criteria when doing a critical appraisal.

After discovering that all SIGN CPGs are developed using the AGREE instrument criteria, one team member browsed the web site of the professional organization, European Society of Cardiology (ESC), that developed the second guideline. The information on ESC's guideline development process that was located did not specify that the AGREE collaboration criteria were used. Therefore, the team conducted a critical appraisal using the AGREE instrument. Team members had to use both the National Guidelines Clearinghouse (NGC) CPG summary and the full-text ESC CPG to appraise the CPG on all 23 AGREE criteria. The team members appraising the CPG scored fifteen of the criteria as 4 (strongly agree), two as 3 (agree), and six as 1 (strongly disagree) because those criteria were not addressed. The six criteria were

- Criterion 5: The patients' views and preferences have been sought.

- Criterion 9: The criteria for selecting the evidence are clearly described.

- Criterion 20: The potential cost implications of applying the recommendations have been considered.

- Criterion 21: The guideline presents key review criteria for monitoring and/or audit purposes.

- Criterion 22: The guideline is editorially independent from the funding body.

- Criterion 23: Conflicts of interest of guideline development members have been recorded.

Despite finding no evidence on which to rate those six criteria, the team judged the ESC CPG to have sufficiently adequate internal validity to inform practice.

Systematic reviews

If the team located a relevant systematic review, its members should use the selected critical appraisal tool to appraise the systematic review's internal validity. If the team members selected a critical appraisal tool that was self-explanatory or that had accompanying instructions, they will have more confidence that they are conducting a rigorous appraisal. An example of a critical appraisal of a systematic review using a slightly modified version of the checklist by SIGN appears in Figure 5-1. After critical appraisal of the systematic review, it was judged to meet all the criteria for internal validity, making it a strong source of evidence for practice.

If the team located more than one systematic review, the members should write a summary that describes the knowledge produced by all of those systematic reviews. This summary will be used later to prepare the synthesis about the knowledge base.

 CASE 5-2 *Summary of Systematic Reviews for the Fabricated Chronic Heart Failure EBP Project*

During the search for systematic reviews, three highly relevant systematic reviews were located. Each is discussed sequentially, followed by a summary of the three systematic reviews.

First, a recent systematic review by McAlister et al.[3] of 29 randomized controlled trials (RCTs) that investigated the effectiveness of multidisciplinary strategies for heart failure patients concluded that the most efficacious strategies were disease management programs that included (1) enhanced patient self-care through patient education, (2) follow-up monitoring by specially trained heart failure (HF) nurses, and (3) access to specialized HF clinics. Programs with follow-up monitoring by specialized multidisciplinary teams, including HF nurses, significantly reduced mortality, HF hospitalizations, and all-cause hospitalizations. Programs that enhanced patient self-care through patient education significantly reduced HF hospitalizations and all-cause hospitalizations, but not mortality. Programs that employed telephone advisement about contacting their primary-care provider if their condition should significantly worsen

Methodology Checklist 1: Systematic Reviews and Meta-analyses	
Title of practice change project: Chronic Heart Failure Management	Team name: Medical EBP Team
PICO Question: P: Chronic heart failure patients I: Long-term management by a nurse practitioner	C: Patient teaching of self-care by a staff nurse O: Unplanned readmission in less than 30 days due to inadequate self-care

Checklist completed by: Jane Doe

Critical appraisal of: McAlister FA, Stewart S, Ferrua S, & McMurray JJ. (2004). Multidisciplinary strategies for the management of heart failure patients at high risk for admission: A systematic review of randomized trials. *J Am Coll Cardiol*, 2004; 44(4): 810-819.

Section 1: Internal validity

In a well-conducted systematic review		In this study, this criterion is	
1.1	The study addresses an appropriate and clearly focused question.	**Well-covered** Adequately addressed Poorly addressed	Not addressed Not reported Not applicable
1.2	A description of the methodology used is included.	**Well-covered** Adequately addressed Poorly addressed	Not addressed Not reported Not applicable
1.3	The literature search is sufficiently rigorous to identify all the relevant studies.	**Well-covered** Adequately addressed Poorly addressed	Not addressed Not reported Not applicable
1.4	Study quality is assessed and taken into account.	**Well-covered** Adequately addressed Poorly addressed	Not addressed Not reported Not applicable

Figure 5-1   Example of a critical appraisal of a systematic review.

1.5	There are enough similarities between the studies selected to make combining them reasonable.	**Well-covered**	Not addressed
		Adequately addressed	Not reported
		Poorly addressed	Not applicable

Section 2: Overall assessment of the study

| 2.1 | **How well was the study done to minimize bias? Code ++, +, or –** | ++ All of the criteria were met. |
| 2.2 | If coded as + or –, what is the likely direction in which bias might affect the study results? | |

Section 3: Description of the study (Please print answers clearly)

3.1	What types of study are included in the review? *(Highlight all that apply)*	**RCT**	CCT	Cohort
		Case control	Other	
3.2	How does this review help to answer your key question? *Summarize the main conclusions of the review and how it relates to the relevant key question. Comment on any particular strengths or weaknesses of the review as a source of evidence for a guideline produced for the NHS in Scotland.*	Review questions were: 1. Can multidisciplinary teams reduce hospitalizations, deaths, and costs? 2. What are the relative benefits of the different interventions? Summary of conclusions: • The most efficacious strategies were disease management programs that included (1) enhanced patient self-care through patient education, (2) follow-up monitoring by specially trained HF nurses, and (3) access to specialized HF clinics. • Programs with follow-up monitoring by specialized multidisciplinary teams, including HF nurses, significantly reduced mortality, HF hospitalizations, and all-cause hospitalizations. • Programs that enhanced patient self-care through patient education significantly reduced HF hospitalizations and all-cause hospitalizations, but not mortality.

Figure 5-1   (*Continued*)

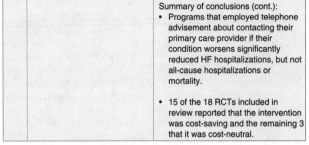

Summary of conclusions (cont.):
- Programs that employed telephone advisement about contacting their primary care provider if their condition worsens significantly reduced HF hospitalizations, but not all-cause hospitalizations or mortality.

- 15 of the 18 RCTs included in review reported that the intervention was cost-saving and the remaining 3 that it was cost-neutral.

Adapted with permission by the Scottish Intercollegiate Guidelines Network (SIGN) from SIGN Methodology Checklist 1

Figure 5-1   (*Continued*)

reduced HF hospitalizations, but not all-cause hospitalizations or mortality. Of the 18 RCTs included in the review, 15 reported that the intervention was cost-saving and the remaining 3 that it was cost-neutral.

Second, a more recent systematic review by Chaudhry et al.[4] of RCTs that investigated the effectiveness of telemonitoring to monitor CHF patients' health status concluded that more evidence is needed about which approaches to telemonitoring are most efficacious and cost-effective. The evidence of effectiveness is heterogeneous. Six of the nine studies reviewed demonstrated reduction in HF hospitalizations, all-cause hospitalizations, and mortality. Three of the nine studies did not demonstrate impact on HF hospitalizations, all-cause hospitalizations, or mortality. For all three of these studies, the reviewers concluded that differences in sample characteristics may have contributed to the discrepant results. Two of those studies included low-risk patients, and one study's sample consisted of high-risk Hispanic CHF patients.

Third, another recent systematic review by Clark et al.[5] examined RCTs that had compared the effectiveness of usual care with telemonitoring or structured telephone support by health professionals, including nurses, and concluded that remote monitoring significantly reduced HF hospitalizations and all-cause mortality. The reviewers observed that telemonitoring and structured telephone support are not treatments and should not be used to replace HF specialist care.

In summary, no systematic reviews were located in which long-term management of CHF was directed by nurse practitioners. Of the three systematic reviews, one[3] of high quality found that multidisciplinary disease management programs that included (1) enhanced patient self-care through patient education, (2) follow-up monitoring by specially trained HF nurses, and (3) access to specialized HF clinics significantly reduced mortality, HF hospitalizations, and all-cause hospitalizations. Furthermore, this one systematic review concluded that programs that enhanced patient self-care through patient education significantly reduced HF hospitalizations and all-cause hospitalizations, but not mortality. There is still limited evidence about the effectiveness of long-term telemonitoring in CHF management. Evidence from all three reviews[3–5] indicates that telemonitoring has the potential to be an effective adjunctive strategy if used in combination with multidisciplinary disease management.

Research

The EBP team members will critically appraise retrieved relevant research reports using the selected data collection tools and checklists. An example of a completed critical appraisal of a quantitative research article appears in Figure 5-2, and an example of a completed critical appraisal of a qualitative research article appears in Figure 5-3. The team should consider having at least two members separately conduct the critical appraisal of their assigned articles using the selected data collection tool, then meet to discuss the similarities and differences in their appraisals. Pairing a member who has some research experience with a member who is a novice at research can be a useful approach to building knowledge of research and the skills for critical appraisal. This approach of pairing can enhance the accuracy and rigor of these critical appraisals. After collecting data about each assigned article, each pair should enter the information into an evidence table. Once all pairs of members have completed their critical appraisals, the team should meet and discuss the evidence from each article. The evidence tables will simplify critical analysis of the effectiveness of the interventions studied.

Citation:	(authors, year, title of article, journal, volume, issue, pages)
	Naylor, MD, et al. Transitional care of older adults hospitalized with heart failure: A randomized, controlled trial. *Journal of the American Geriatrics Society*. 2004; 52(5): 675-684.[8]

Aims, research questions, or hypotheses:	To examine the effectiveness of a transitional care intervention delivered by advanced practice nurses (APNs) to elders

Type:	X	Quantitative		Mixed methods

Study site:	6 Philadelphia academic and community hospitals

Sample:	Size: 239 patients	Sampling plan: Random assignment
	Demographics: aged 65 or older; mean age 76; 43% male; 36% African American	

Variables and instruments	Dependent:	- Rehospitalization or death - Total costs - Hospital days - Quality of life - Satisfaction with care
	Independent:	Transitional care intervention delivered by advanced practice nurses (APNs)
	Confounding:	NA due to sampling plan

Design	Experimental		Nonexperimental
	X	Randomized controlled trial		Cohort study
		Experiment		Case control study
		Quasi-experimental		Descriptive comparative study
				Descriptive correlation study
				Descriptive exploratory study

| Results: | Compared to control group, intervention group had:

- Longer time to first rehospitalization or death (log rank χ^2 = 5.0, p = .026)

-Fewer readmissions (104 vs. 162, p = .047)

-Lower mean total costs ($7,636 vs. $12, 481)

-Fewer rehospitalizations (22 of 104) related to comorbidities than did the control group (50 of 162) |
|---|---|

Figure 5-2 Example of a completed appraisal of a quantitative research article. (*Continued*)

	-Fewer hospital days (588) than the control group (970, p = .071)	
	-Higher quality of life (Minnesota Living with Heart Failure Questionnaire) at 12 weeks (p <.05)	
	-Higher satisfaction with care at 2 weeks and 6 weeks (p <.001)	
	-At 52 weeks, had lower mean total costs of care, including the intervention cost	
Recommendations:	APN-directed transitional care for heart failure may be effective in increasing length of time before hospitalization or death, reduced total number of hospitalizations, and reduced costs of care in other urban hospitals in the U.S.	
Strengths:	Internal validity:	External validity:
	-APNs coordinated care related to all comorbidities that could affect stability of clinical condition	May be generalizable to other major U.S. cities
	-Sample size large enough to detect differences between groups	
	-Thorough explanation of how missing data were handled to avoid loss of participants during analyses	
	-6 sites	
Limitations:	Internal validity:	External validity:
		May not be generalizable to rural patients
	ANALYSIS	
Clinical significance:	Highly significant because of current poor CHF management outcomes	
Credibility of results:	Very credible because of excellent internal validity	
Intervention applicable to my setting:	Questionable—could we recruit nurse practitioners to our rural setting? Would it be as effective with our rural patients?	
Acceptability of benefit vs. risk:	Excellent evidence of benefit with no perceptible risks	
Acceptability of costs:	Yes, lower cost than usual care	

Figure 5-2 (*Continued*)

Literature Review Worksheet Qualitative Research

Citation: (authors, year, title of article, journal, volume, issue, pages)
Schnell, KN, Naimark, BJ, and McClement, SE. Influential factors for self-care in ambulatory care heart failure patients: A qualitative perspective. *Canadian Journal of Cardiovascular Nursing.* 2006; 16(1):13-19.[10]

Purpose, aims, or research questions: To describe the influences that enhance or impede self-care and to explore behavioral responses to these influences.

Research tradition:
Content analysis ___X___ Grounded theory _____ Ethnography _____ Mixed methods _____ Other _____
Used a semi-structured interview for data collection, using an interview guide based on Connelly's Model of Self-Care in Chronic Illness.

Study site: A Manitoba, Canada community

Sample:
   Size: _11_   Sampling plan: _Purposive_   Demographics: 7 men; 10 Caucasian, 1 Aboriginal; mean age of 64, range 43
– 79; 6 lived inside city limits, 5 lived outside city limits; all recruited from a CHF management clinic

Phenomenon of interest: Facilitators and barriers of self-care by persons with CHF

Results: Patients were more self-care compliant when they
- were satisfied with their clinic care,
- had positive attitudes towards their health,
- had positive family support,
- recognized their own role responsibilities for self-care,
- were able to recognize heart failure symptoms that required their taking action,
- did not perceive self-care strategies to threaten their self-concept, and
- perceived that the self-care strategies offered more benefit than burden.

Figure 5-3 Example of a critical appraisal of a qualitative research article.

A couple of patients did not know they had the option of calling the clinic about their heart failure symptoms and one patient thought that it was the responsibility of the health-care provider to call them to evaluate their health status.

Recommendations: Nurses should individualize the self-care teaching plan and should monitor CHF patient's health status through regular telephone contact.

Appraisal questions:
Did researcher report preconceptions or biases? Not explicitly; however, by basing the interview guide on a theoretical model precluded the researcher from discovering any concepts not already in that model.
Was the research tradition appropriate for the purpose of the study? Yes
If there was a theoretical framework, was it appropriate for the research tradition? Acceptable
Were the data collection procedures appropriate for the research tradition? Yes
Were included informants appropriate for the purpose of the study? Yes
Did data collection continue until redundancy or data saturation was reached? Not discussed explicitly but the 11 patients were recruited before the study began and any analysis, suggesting that data saturation was not an aim.
Is analysis described with sufficient detail that another researcher could replicate the study? Yes
Is the description of results appropriate for the research tradition? Yes
Does the discussion include linkages of results to existing knowledge? Yes, to other research findings. Could have also discussed that the findings provide empirical support for the concepts in Connelly's Model of Self-Care in Chronic Illness.

Figure 5-3 (Continued)

Trustworthiness

Credibility: Acceptable. The sampling plan was adequate to obtain appropriate informants about CHF self-care. The data and results were examined by an experienced qualitative researcher and verified. There was no mention of conducting "member checks," sharing results and obtaining feedback from some of the informants, which is a limitation.

Dependability: Acceptable. The description of the design and procedures was sufficient for another researcher to replicate the study.

Confirmability: Acceptable. The findings appear to reflect the informants' experience, as evidenced by the verbatim quotations from informants.

Transferability: Acceptable. Although the author did not provide a full description of the context in which the study was conducted, some of the findings reflected the influence of the informants' home context.

ANALYSIS

Clinical significance: Highly clinically significant because of the consequences to the patient, family, health-care system, and society of poor self-care by persons with CHF.

Intervention applicable to my setting: It is potentially applicable if organization leaders will prepare nurses to be experts in CHF and teaching self-care.

Acceptability of benefit vs. risk: Yes. Implementing the suggested recommendations has the potential to improve CHF self-care and reduce avoidable hospitalizations.

Acceptability of costs: No cost analysis was included in the study. However, the cost of providing avoidable hospital care to patients with CHF is quite high, making it worth exploring implementing the suggested recommendations.

Figure 5-3 (Continued)

CASE 5-3 *Evidence Tables for the Fabricated CHF EBP Project*

The EBP team limited its search for research reports to the past five years because of the availability of two systematic reviews with strong internal validity and two CPGs with good internal validity. Many relevant research reports published in the past five years were located, including RCTs. Therefore, the team limited the evidence presented in its first evidence table (Figure 5-4) to RCTs, because they have

Author, Date	Aims, Research Questions, or Hypotheses	Methodology: Design, Site, Sample	Intervention	Results	Strengths and Limitations
Koelling, Johnson, Cody, & Aaronson, 2005[7]	To compare effectiveness of a 1-hour, one-to-one teaching session with usual care	-RCT with follow-up data collected at 30, 90, and 180 days post discharge -223 heart failure patients, mean age 65, 42% female, 22% (control group) and 21% (intervention group) African American -One academic medical center in Michigan	Standard care plus 1- hour, one-to-one teaching session by a nurse educator, plus copy of treatment guidelines prior to discharge	-Intervention group had fewer days hospitalized or dead within the follow-up period (0 and 10 days, $p = .009$) than did control group (4 and 19 days) at 180 days post-intervention -Scores on 6 self-care behaviors were higher at 30 days post discharge for patients in the intervention group and were significantly higher for three of the six behaviors: weighing daily, following sodium restriction, and not smoking. -Cost of care including cost of the intervention, were lower for the intervention group than control group by $2823 per patient ($p = .035$)	Strengths -RCT, with care providers and patient blinded to group assignment Limitations - Data collector not blinded to group assignment - Self-report on self-care behaviors - Adequacy of sample size not discussed - Urban setting only, possibly not generalizable to rural patients

Figure 5-4   Example of a table of evidence from quantitative research studies for the fabricated CHF project. (*Continued*)

| Kimmelstiel et al., 2004[6] | To evaluate the effectiveness of a nurse-led heart failure disease management program | -RCT

-200 patients with heart failure patients, mean age 70.3 (intervention group) and 73.9 (control); 42% female

-6 sites including academic medical centers, community hospitals, and community cardiac practices | -90-day post discharge disease management led by HF-experienced nurse managers

-Home visit with individualized teaching and printed educational material

-Received contact information of assigned nurse and for a 24-hour on-call nurse

-Assigned nurse:

-Telephoned patients weekly or biweekly to reinforce education

-Had 24-hour on-call access to HF physicians

-Communicated patient condition frequently to primary-care providers, providing recommendations of regimen changes made by HF physicians | -Intervention group had fewer HF hospitalizations (0.55) than control group (1.14, $p = 0.27$)

-Intervention group had fewer hospital days (4.3) than control group (7.8, $p = <.001$)

-Most gain lost by 180 days post intervention | Strengths
- Design

- Data collectors were blinded to group assignment

Limitations
- Consistency of intervention by nurse managers not discussed

- Urban settings only, possibly not generalizable to rural patients |
| Naylor et al., 2004[8] | To examine the effectiveness of a transitional care intervention delivered by advanced practice nurses (APNs) to elders hospitalized with heart failure | -RCT, with post-discharge follow-up for 52 weeks

-239 patients aged 65 or older; mean age 76; 43% male; 36% African American

-6 Philadelphia academic and community hospitals | A 3-month APN-directed discharge planning and home follow-up protocol plus printed educational material | Compared to control group, intervention group had:

- Longer time to first rehospitalization or death (log rank $\chi^2 = 5.0$, $p = .026$)

-Fewer readmissions (104 vs. 162, $p = .047$)

-Lower mean total costs ($7,636 vs. $12,481) | Strengths
-Strongest design

-APNs coordinated care related to all comorbidities that could affect stability of clinical condition

-Sample size large enough to detect differences between groups

-Thorough explanation of how missing data were handled to avoid loss of participants during analyses |

Figure 5-4   (*Continued*)

Naylor et al., 2004[B] (Cont.)				-Fewer rehospitalizations (22 of 104) related to co-morbidities than did the control group (50 of 162)	-6 sites Limitations -Urban settings only, possibly not generalizable to rural patients
				-Fewer hospital days (588) than control group (970, $p = .071$)	
				-Higher quality of life (Minnesota Living with Heart Failure Questionnaire) at 12 weeks ($p <.05$). Higher satisfaction with care at 2 weeks and 6 weeks ($p <.001$)	

Figure 5-4   (*Continued*)

stronger internal validity than other research designs. The team searched for qualitative research studies about CHF self-care. No relevant phenomenology, grounded theory, or ethnographic studies were located. The data for the two relevant studies that did content analysis appear in the second evidence table (Figure 5-5).

Weighing the Validity and Strength of the Evidence

In addition to making judgments about the effectiveness of the interventions, the team makes judgments about the internal validity of all the evidence to determine the strength of the evidence. Systematic reviews with excellent internal validity provide the strongest evidence for practice (Figure 5-1). Clinical practice guidelines with excellent internal validity also provide good evidence for practice because they are based on systematic reviews, and their recommendations are labeled to indicate the strength of the evidence supporting each one. Randomized controlled trials provide the strongest evidence of intervention effectiveness of any research design.

Citation	Purpose, Aims, or Research Questions	Methodology: Design, Site, Sample	Results	Strengths and Limitations
Schnell et al., 2006[10]	To describe the influences that enhance or impede self-care and to explore behavioral responses to these influences	• Content analysis of data collected using semi-structured interview guide • A Manitoba, Canada community • 11 CHF patients • 7 men, 4 women • 10 Caucasian, 1 Aboriginal • 6 lived inside and 5 lived outside city limits	Patients were more self-care compliant when they • were satisfied with their clinic care, • had positive attitudes towards their health, • had positive family support, • recognized their own role responsibilities for self-care, • were able to recognize heart failure symptoms that required their taking action, • did not perceive self-care strategies to threaten their self concept, and • perceived that the self-care strategies offered more benefit than burden.	Met most of the characteristics of trustworthiness
Riegel & Carlson, 2002[11]	To explore the impact of HF on patients' lives, assess their self-care behaviors, and determine how their life situations facilitate or impede heart failure self-care	• Content analysis of data collected using a structured interview guide • Large health-care system in southern California • 26 CHF patients • 17 men, 9 women • Mean age = 74.4+ 10.05 years	Three themes emerged: 1. Facing the challenges of living with heart failure: • Physical limitations • Difficulty coping with treatment • Lack of knowledge or misconceptions • Distressed emotions • Multiple comorbidities • Personal struggles 2. Performing self-care • Symptom recognition • Following the treatment regimen 3. Finding ways to adapt • Practical adaptations • Learning about heart failure • Maintaining control • Depending on others • Ignoring, withdrawing, accepting	Met most of the characteristics of trustworthiness

Figure 5-5   Example of a table of evidence from qualitative research studies for the fabricated CHF project.

Based on the team's critical appraisal of the internal validity of the individual evidence documents, members can make a judgment about the strength of the evidence for the collective body of evidence appraised. This is done by examining the evidence tables and comparing them with the hierarchy of research designs in Figure 4-1.

SYNTHESIZE THE BEST EVIDENCE

Having completed the critical appraisal of the evidence and weighed the internal validity and strength of the evidence, the EBP team next writes the synthesis using the summarized evidence from systematic reviews and CPGs and the evidence tables about research. Figure 5-6 displays an example of using the synthesis worksheet template (Figure 4-10) to prepare the content for the narrative synthesis. The focus of the synthesis is on the evidence, not the producers of the evidence. First, the team writes clear, concise statements about the findings that are supported by the evidence, citing the supportive evidence. These statements are the state of the science of the reviewed knowledge base. The synthesis should address whether the evidence is homogeneous (consistent) or heterogeneous (inconsistent). If the evidence is heterogeneous, the synthesis should contain plausible explanations for the inconsistencies. To accomplish that, the team should include a critical analysis of the strength of the evidence, which is accomplished by analyzing threats to the internal validity of the studies. Based on that critical analysis, the synthesis also comments on the strength of the body of evidence. Finally, the synthesis should identify gaps in the knowledge base about the topic and make specific recommendations for future research to address those gaps.

Having written the synthesis of the evidence, the EBP team makes a judgment about whether or not the evidence supports a practice change. Should the evidence be judged to be too weak or inconclusive, the team will decide that the evidence does not support a practice change. In this case, the team will end its work on that project. Should the team judge that the evidence is sufficiently strong to support a practice change, the team then considers the feasibility, benefits, and risks of the proposed practice change.

Synthesis Worksheet
A. Write clear, concise statements about the findings that are supported by the evidence and identify the supportive evidence.
1. Two CPGs,[1,2] one systematic review,[3] and three RCTs[6-8] strongly support the effectiveness of patient teaching and long-term follow-up in reducing hospitalizations and costs and in delaying death.
2. Multidisciplinary disease management programs, including HF-specialist nurses involved in teaching and follow-up were more effective than either usual care or HF-specialist teaching, at time of discharge only, in achieving the desired outcomes.[3,7]
3. HF specialist teaching at time of discharge only was more effective than usual care.[7]
4. One strong RCT[8] with long-term management directed by advanced nurse practitioners (APN) was more effective than usual care.
5. Telemonitoring may be a useful adjunct to multidisciplinary disease management.[4,5]
6. Two qualitative studies[10,11] supported assessment of the patient's motivation and facilitators and barriers to CHF self-care before initiating an individualized teaching plan.
B. Write statements regarding whether the body of evidence is homogeneous (consistent) or heterogeneous (inconsistent).
1. The evidence of the effectiveness of patient teaching and long-term follow-up in reducing hospitalizations and costs and in delaying death was homogeneous.
2. According to two systematic reviews of RCTs,[4,5] the evidence of the effectiveness of telemonitoring as an adjunct to multidisciplinary disease management is predominately, but not entirely, homogeneous.
3.

Figure 5-6 Example of a completed synthesis worksheet. (*Continued*)

	Synthesis Worksheet (Cont.)
C.	If the body of evidence is heterogeneous (inconsistent), write explicit statements regarding plausible explanations for the inconsistencies. (Tip: They are usually due to how well the design of a study is controlled for threats to internal validity; to a sample size that is too small to have enough power to detect an intervention's effect or a difference; or to noncomparable sample characteristics. You would usually have more confidence in studies designed to control for threats to internal validity with adequate sample sizes than in other studies.)
1.	According to one systematic review[4], three studies that failed to demonstrate effectiveness of telemonitoring of community-dwelling CHF patients had nonrepresentative samples: two enrolled low-risk patients and one enrolled very high-risk Hispanic patients.
2.	
3.	
D.	Write clear, explicit statements about the remaining gaps in the knowledge base.
1.	Further research is needed before recommending telemonitoring as an adjunct to multidisciplinary disease management.[4]
2.	Further research is needed to validate the effectiveness of long-term management directed by APNs compared to usual care, especially in rural patients receiving care in their own communities.
3.	
E.	Based on your critical analysis of the evidence, write conclusions regarding the adequacy of the evidence to support a practice change.
1.	There was sufficient evidence to support a practice change to the existing multidisciplinary disease management program by adding the component of nurses specialized in CHF assessment and teaching who would be responsible for long-term telephone follow-up of CHF patients.
2.	
3.	

Figure 5-6 (*Continued*)

CASE 5-4 *Synthesis for the Fabricated CHF EBP Project*

Evidence from internally valid CPGs,[1,2] two systematic reviews,[3–5] and RCTs[6–8] strongly supports the effectiveness of patient teaching and long-term follow-up in reducing hospitalizations and costs and in delaying death. Multidisciplinary disease management programs, including involving HF specialist nurses in teaching and follow-up, were more effective in achieving the desired outcomes than either usual care or HF specialist teaching at the time of discharge only.[3,7] Also, HF specialist teaching at the time of discharge only was more effective than usual care.[7] There is evidence from one strong RCT[8] that long-term management directed by advanced nurse practitioners (APN) was more effective than usual care. However, further evidence is needed to corroborate the findings of this RCT, especially using samples of rural patients receiving care in their own communities. Telemonitoring may be a useful adjunct to multidisciplinary disease management, but further research is needed before recommending its addition.[4,5] According to one systematic review,[4] three studies that failed to demonstrate the effectiveness of telemonitoring of community-dwelling CHF patients had nonrepresentative samples: two enrolled low-risk patients, and one enrolled very high risk Hispanic patients. Finally, the findings of the two qualitative studies reviewed (Figure 5-5) supported assessment of the patient's motivation and facilitators and barriers to CHF self-care before initiating an individualized teaching plan. The EBP team concluded that there was sufficient evidence to support a practice change to the existing multidisciplinary disease management program by adding the component of nurses specializing in CHF assessment and teaching who would be responsible for long-term telephone follow-up of CHF patients, including assessment of the patient's motivation and facilitators and barriers to CHF self-care before initiating an individualized teaching plan.

ASSESS THE FEASIBILITY, BENEFITS, AND RISK OF THE NEW PRACTICE

Having synthesized the best evidence and concluding that it supported a practice change, the EBP team describes the evidence-based content of the proposed new practice, including any structure characteristics and the process. The description of the proposed new practice should reflect the practice that was investigated in evidence documents. Based on that description, the team can consider the feasibility of implementing the new practice in its setting. There is evidence[9] that a new practice is more likely to be accepted if it is a good "fit" with the organization. Team members who understand their own organization are able to judge the fit.

Simultaneously with judging the feasibility of the new practice, the EBP team should consider the benefits and risks of implementing the new practice. Will the benefits outweigh any risks to the patient? If there are any risks of implementing the new practice, are they sufficiently minor that they are acceptable? Are there any organizational, time, or cost challenges in implementing the new practice? There is evidence[9] that a new practice is more likely to be adopted if it has obvious benefits to the patient that are better than those provided by the current practice. If the benefits are marginal or the anticipated costs are high, the EBP team is likely to decide that the new practice is not worth the investment of time and money required to implement it. When a team decides that a new practice is supported by the evidence and is feasible, with potential benefits and acceptable costs, its members should obtain patient or family member feedback on the proposed practice change before moving into Step 4 of the EBP model.

 CASE 5-5 *Summary of Evidence-Based Teaching Content for CHF Patients*

Teach patients and family the following and reinforce it long-term:

• Weight monitoring.
  — Weigh oneself daily after waking and voiding and before dressing and eating.

— If there is an unexpected weight gain of >2 kg in 3 days, call the health-care provider or follow the guidelines provided to adjust the diuretic dose.

- Dietary measures.
  — Sodium.
    - Avoid salt intake >6 g/day.
    - Avoid "low salt" substitutes.
  — Fluids.
    - Individualize fluid restriction.
    - Restrict to 1.5 to 2 L/day if in advanced heart failure.
  — Alcohol.
    - Limit to moderate alcohol intake (one beer, one to two glasses of wine/day).
    - Stop drinking alcohol if have alcoholic cardiomyopathy.
  — Obesity.
    - Lose weight if obese.
- Smoking.
  — Stop smoking.
  — Use smoking cessation aids, including nicotine replacement therapies.
- Exercise.
  — Engage in regular, low-intensity exercise, with health-care provider approval.

 CASE 5-6 *Decision about the Feasibility, Benefits, and Risks of the New Practice for the Fabricated CHF Project*

The EBP team considered the feasibility, benefits, and risks of adding to the existing multidisciplinary disease management program the component of nurses specializing in CHF assessing and teaching who would be responsible for long-term telephone follow-up of CHF patients. Team members knew that there were nurses at the hospital who were interested in working with CHF patients and who would probably be willing to obtain specialized education in assessing CHF patients and teaching them CHF self-care. By regular telephone monitoring of CHF patients, the CHF nurse specialists would be able to reinforce the patients' knowledge about self-care, potentially reducing exacerbations of CHF symptoms and hospitalizations. The team judged that the reduced number of CHF hospitalizations would offset the costs associated with having two nurses in a full-time position as CHF nurse specialists. The only patients who would not benefit from the new practice would be those rural and impoverished patients who had no telephone. Although this was not an intervention that was evaluated in any of the evidence, the team decided to add a trial use of mailed postcards for patients without telephones to allow them to mail back answers to simple health status assessment questions. With this addition, the team decided that the new practice was feasible and had potential benefits and acceptable costs and moved on to Step 4.

REFERENCES

1. Scottish Intercollegiate Guidelines Network (SIGN). Management of chronic heart failure: A national clinical guideline. February 2007; available through the National Guidelines Clearinghouse, http://www.guideline.gov/. Accessed July 19, 2007.

2. Swedberg K, Cleland J, Dargie H, et al. Guidelines for the diagnosis and treatment of chronic heart failure. 2005; available through the National Guidelines Clearinghouse, http://www.guideline.gov/. Accessed July 19, 2007.

3. McAlister FA, Stewart S, Ferrua S, McMurray JJ. Multidisciplinary strategies for the management of heart failure patients at high risk for admission: A systematic review of randomized trials. *J Am Coll Cardiol*. Aug 18 2004;44(4):810–819.

4. Chaudhry SI, Phillips CO, Stewart SS, et al. Telemonitoring for patients with chronic heart failure: A systematic review. *J Card Fail*. Feb 2007;13(1):56–62.

5. Clark RA, Inglis SC, McAlister FA, et al. Telemonitoring or structured telephone support programmes for patients with chronic heart failure: Systematic review and meta-analysis. *BMJ*. May 5 2007;334(7600):942.

6. Kimmelstiel C, Levine D, Perry K, et al. Randomized, controlled evaluation of short- and long-term benefits of heart failure disease management within a diverse provider network: The SPAN-CHF trial. *Circulation*. Sep 14 2004; 110(11):1450–1455.

7. Koelling TM, Johnson ML, Cody RJ, Aaronson KD. Discharge education improves clinical outcomes in patients with chronic heart failure. *Circulation*. Jan 18 2005;111(2):179–185.

8. Naylor MD, Brooten DA, Campbell RL, et al. Transitional care of older adults hospitalized with heart failure: A randomized, controlled trial. *J Am Geriatr Soc*. 2004;52(5):675–684.

9. Greenhalgh T, Robert G, Macfarlane F, et al. Diffusion of innovations in service organizations: Systematic review and recommendations. *Milbank Q*. 2004;82(4):581–629.

10. Schnell KN, Naimark BJ, McClement SE. Influential factors for self-care in ambulatory care heart failure patients: A qualitative perspective. *Can J Cardiovasc Nurs*. 2006;16(1):13–19.

11. Riegel B, Carlson B. Facilitators and barriers to heart failure self-care. *Patient Educ Couns*. Apr 2002;46(4):287–295.

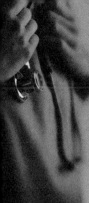

Chapter 6
STEP 4: DESIGN PRACTICE CHANGE

- **DEFINE THE PROPOSED CHANGE**
  - —Identify Process Variables
  - —Key Attributes of the New Practice
- **IDENTIFY NEEDED RESOURCES**
  - —Identify Structure Variables
- **DESIGN THE EVALUATION OF THE PILOT**
  - —Identify Outcome Variables
  - —Develop the Evaluation Plan
- **DESIGN THE IMPLEMENTATION PLAN**
  - —Design the Pilot Study
    - *Select pilot sites*
    - *Enhance adoption of the new practice by stakeholders*
    - *Decide on the time interval for the pilot*
    - *Design the plan for monitoring the fidelity of the pilot*
    - *Design the marketing plan*
    - *Assign responsibilities and plan timelines*
  - —Obtain Agency Approvals for Pilot
  - —Prepare Pilot Sites

In this step, the evidence-based practice (EBP) team defines the proposed practice change and identifies the resources needed for nurses to perform the new practice. Then the team designs the evaluation plan and the implementation plan.

DEFINE THE PROPOSED CHANGE

Identify Process Variables

The EBP team must develop a document that describes the details of the new practice. The format may be a procedure, policy, care map, or guideline, whichever is preferred by the nursing leadership. The content describes which patients the practice pertains to, the processes of care, the appropriate timing of the processes, and the expected documentation. The description of the new practice must include only processes that were evaluated in the evidence base. Also, relevant patients must be similar to those included in the evidence base.

Key Attributes of the New Practice

Evidence indicates that an innovation, such as a new practice, is more likely to be adopted if it possesses these five key *attributes* that research indicates are critical for successful implementation of a new practice:

* Relative advantage
* Observable benefits
* Simplicity
* "Augmented support" for technology
* Innovation/system fit

New practices that are viewed as having a clear relative advantage over alternative approaches in terms of observable benefits (effectiveness or cost-effectiveness)[1–5] and for which the risks are perceived as minimal relative to the benefits are more readily implemented.[3,6] Organization members are more likely to implement new practices that they perceive as having simplicity (minimal complexity); that is, they can be viewed as having smaller, more manageable components or can be implemented in stages.[2–4,6–8] When the new practice involves new technology, provision of augmented support for the use of that technology has been shown to enhance its adoption.[5,9] For instance, implementing the use of a bladder scanner to reduce nosocomial urinary tract infections associated with catheterization requires demonstration and instruction in the use of the bladder scanner.[10] Finally, designing a new practice (innovation) so that it fits the organization (innovation/system fit) is critical to successful implementation.[3,4,7,11] The members of the EBP team should consider this evidence about key attributes as they define the new practice.

IDENTIFY NEEDED RESOURCES

Identify Structure Variables

As the EBP team members define the new practice, they need to consider what resources will be needed to enable nurses to perform the new practice. First, they need to determine the nurse role that will be expected to perform the care. The nurse role may be the registered nurse (RN), licensed practical nurse, nursing assistant, or a specialty role, such as a clinical nurse specialist, wound care and ostomy nurse, or intravenous therapy nurse.

Second, the nature of the new practice may require the team to develop or obtain special materials. These may include patient and family education materials and fact sheets. A number of these are available online or in print. Web sites with patient educational resources include:

- Medline Plus—Interactive Health Tutorials: http://www.nlm.nih.gov/medlineplus/tutorial.html
- American Diabetes Association: http://www.diabetes.org/home.jsp
- American Cancer Society: http://www.cancer.org/docroot/home/index.asp

- American Lung Association: http://www.lungusa.org/site/pp.asp?c=dvLUK9O0E&b=22542
- American Heart Association: http://www.americanheart.org/presenter.jhtml?identifier=1200000
- American College of Rheumatology: http://www.rheumatology.org/public/factsheets/index.asp
- Ohio State University Medical Center: Patient Education Materials: http://medicalcenter.osu.edu/patientcare/patient_education/
- Journal of the American Medical Association—JAMA Patient Page: http://jama.ama-assn.org/cgi/collection/patient_page
- Ohio State University—Patient Education Resources for Clinicians: http://www.ohsu.edu/library/patiented/links.shtml
- University of California, San Francisco—Patient Education: http://www.ucsfhealth.org/adult/edu/

To locate existing patient education materials, a team member could perform an Internet browser search using as search words "patient education" and "name of the condition," such as "diabetes," "cancer," or "chronic heart failure." However, the team may be unable to locate an existing educational resource that is relevant to the new practice and so may need to develop one.

Third, some new practices will require the use of equipment. For instance, using a bladder scanner to reduce the incidence of urinary tract infections requires availability of a bladder scanner, which is a capital equipment expense.[10] As another example, postoperative wound dressing changes require the use of sterile gloves, a relatively minor expense when compared to the costs associated with postoperative wound infections.[12]

Fourth, the team must consider the need for developing any new forms that would support the nurse's use of the new practice. Experience indicates that providing instructions about using existing documentation forms is more acceptable to direct-care nurses than introducing a new form, especially if a new form requires duplicating some documentation elements. However, there are instances where existing forms are inadequate for documenting the performance of a new practice.

Case 6-1 *Child Visitation in the Cardiothoracic/Coronary Care Unit*

The Critical Care EBP Team at West Virginia University Hospitals (WVUH) conducted a project to increase family presence for critically ill persons, with a focus on allowing children under 14 years of age to visit a hospitalized parent or grandparent.[13] Based on the evidence that its members critically appraised, the team developed a revised child visitation policy that allowed children over 12 months of age to visit a parent, grandparent, or great-grandparent for 5 to 15 minutes. Implementation activities were:

- Provided formal education of RNs and support staff.
- Developed an information letter to parents about the child visitation policy.
- Prepared a health screening packet to assess the suitability of allowing a visit, for the safety of both the child and the critically ill family member.
- Created an intensive care unit (ICU) coloring book to help desensitize children to the sights common in an ICU.
- Purchased child-size rocking chairs for children to use while visiting.
- Purchased stickers to give to children after the visit is completed.
- Prepared a prepaid postcard for parents to use after the visit to comment on the visitation experience for their family.

DESIGN THE EVALUATION OF THE PILOT

The ultimate aim of an EBP change is to improve outcomes for patients. The EBP team may include as project goals the achievement of other outcomes pertaining to patients' families, staff, other disciplines, organization leaders, and costs. To judge an EBP project's achievement of the desired outcomes, the team must identify the target outcome variables and develop an evaluation plan.

Identify Outcome Variables

The evidence that was synthesized during Step 3 focused on specific outcomes that were either desired outcomes of care or undesired outcomes to be avoided. Desired outcomes are positive consequences of care. The team would anticipate improvement from the baseline measure of such outcomes to the postpilot measure. Examples of desired outcomes include adequate cardiac function, cognitive orientation, pain control, activity tolerance, wound healing, and patient satisfaction. In the fabricated chronic heart failure (CHF) EBP project, two desired outcomes were *improved self-care* and *reduced costs associated with avoidable CHF-related rehospitalizations*.

Undesired outcomes are adverse consequences of care. The team would anticipate reduction in the postpilot measure compared to the baseline measure of such outcomes. Examples of undesired outcomes include nosocomial infection, elopement, falls, hemorrhage, aspiration, and wrong amputation. In the fabricated CHF EBP project, the team anticipated that the new practice would reduce the rate of CHF-related rehospitalizations, an undesired outcome. Team members will identify the outcome variables for their EBP project from the evidence synthesized in Step 3.

Develop the Evaluation Plan

Having identified the process and outcome variables for the new practice, the team develops the evaluation plan. If the process and outcome variables remain the same as those used to collect internal data about the problem during Step 1, the evaluation plan will consist of using the same data collection instrument (DCI), arranging to collect the postpilot data, and comparing the baseline data with the postpilot data. However, if the process and outcome variables have changed, the EBP team will need to design a new DCI that includes rate-based indicators or measures of those variables, collect baseline data before initiating the pilot, and plan to collect the postpilot data and to compare the baseline data with the postpilot data.

As mentioned in Step 1, the team must also decide on the sample size. The Joint Commission on Accreditation of Healthcare Organizations (the Joint Commission)[14, p. HM-8] requires the following sample sizes when collecting data about structure or process elements of a standard of care. These sample categories may be used when deciding on a sample size for the EBP project evaluation:

- "for a population of
  — fewer than 30 cases, sample 100% of available cases
  — 30 to 100 cases, sample 30 cases
  — 101 to 500 cases, sample 50 cases
  — greater than 500 cases, sample 70 cases"

For greater confidence that the size will be adequate, the team should consider using sample size calculator software. There are a number of web sites that provide access to statistical software. One web site that includes sample size calculators is http://statpages.org/.

There are introductory statistics books available should members of an EBP team wish to begin developing an understanding of statistics, including sample size calculation.[15,16] Some health-care organizations may have a decision support department that can perform the sample size calculation. If the team plans to conduct the evaluation component of the project as a research study, it should consult with someone who has statistical expertise about the appropriate sample size. If there is no resource person in the organization who can perform the power analysis, the EBP team should explore the possibility of finding a statistician to serve as a consultant. One approach would be to browse the web site of the department of statistics or department of mathematics at a local or regional university. Once the team knows the target sample size, it needs to estimate, based on volume, the length of time that will be required to obtain that number. This estimate will indicate the length of time needed to complete the data collection portion of the evaluation.

Case 6-2 *Defining the Process, Structure, and Outcome Variables for the Fabricated CHF Practice Change*

In Case 5-4, the EBP team for the fabricated CHF project concluded that there was sufficient evidence to support a practice change to the existing multidisciplinary disease management program by adding the component of nurses specializing in CHF assessment and teaching who would be responsible for long-term telephone follow-up of CHF patients, including assessment of the patient's motivation and facilitators and barriers to CHF self-care before initiating an individualized teaching plan. In Case 5-5, the team itemized the evidence-based teaching content needed by CHF patients, and in Case 5-6, the team summarized the feasibility and benefits of adding two CHF nurse specialists and phone monitoring and follow-up education to the existing CHF disease management program. Because of the thoroughness of that work in Step 3, the team, in Step 4, identified the process variables as

- Referral of CHF patients by staff nurses for evaluation by the CHF nurse specialists within 24 hours of a CHF admission
- Assessment by the CHF nurse specialists of the patient's motivation and facilitators and barriers to CHF self-care
- Evaluation of health status and CHF self-care knowledge by the CHF nurse specialists
- Individualized teaching about CHF self-care by the CHF nurse specialists
- Biweekly telephone follow-up about health status and CHF self-care knowledge by the CHF nurse specialist

Based on the evidence summarized in Cases 5-2 to 5-5, the team identified the following structure variables:

- Extensive educational preparation of the two RNs who were selected to become the CHF nurse specialists
- Office space with telephones and computers for both CHF nurse specialists
- Permission to use the Self-Care of Heart Failure Index (SCHFI)[17]
- Patient educational resources

The team identified a number of patient educational resources that the CHF specialist nurses could choose from when individualizing teaching, including the CHF patient resources at these sites:

- Medline Plus—Interactive Health Tutorials: http://www.nlm.nih.gov/medlineplus/tutorial.html
- American Heart Association: http://www.americanheart.org/presenter.jhtml?identifier=1200000
- Heart Point: http://www.heartpoint.com/
- Heart Failure Online: http://www.heartfailure.org/
- Mayo Clinic—Heart Failure: http://www.mayoclinic.com/health/heart-failure/DS00061/UPDATEAPP=0

Based on the evidence summarized in Cases 5-2 to 5-5, the team identified the following outcome variables:

- Increase CHF patients' mean scores on the Self-Care of Heart Failure Index[17] at six months post-CHF hospitalization by 10 percent.
- Reduce the CHF readmission rate at six months post-CHF hospitalization by 10 percent.

The team incorporated the process, structure, and outcome variables in a description of the new practice in the format of a policy.

DESIGN THE IMPLEMENTATION PLAN

In designing the implementation plan, the EBP team will design the pilot study, obtain agency approvals for the pilot study, and prepare the pilot sites. Designing the pilot study consists of selecting the pilot sites, deciding on the time interval for the pilot, planning the timelines, designing the marketing plan, designing the plan for monitoring the fidelity of the pilot, and assigning responsibilities for conducting the pilot.

Design the Pilot Study

Select pilot sites

Some new practices will be relevant to more than one nursing unit, such as the medical-surgical and adult intensive care units, while others will be relevant to only one unique unit, such as a neonatal intensive care unit. Regardless, the EBP team should consider the initial implementation of the new practice as a pilot phase and communicate that perspective to stakeholders of the new practice. When the new practice is relevant to more than one nursing unit, the EBP team must decide whether to pilot the new practice on just one unit or all relevant units. Simplicity is an advantage of piloting the new practice on just one of the relevant units because fewer nurses are required to participate in conducting the pilot. Representation is an advantage of piloting the new practice on all relevant units because all stakeholders will have an opportunity to give the EBP team members their opinions and suggestions about the new practice during the pilot phase.

Enhance adoption of the innovation by individuals

Considerable research has identified several strategies for enhancing the adoption of innovations, such as new practices, by individuals. These strategies include:

• Representation and participation
• Education
• Use of social networks (opinion leaders and change champions)
• Performance feedback

First, when the decision to adopt a new practice is participative, rather than authoritative,[4,18,19] and when persons perceive that they have the autonomy and the opportunity to adapt or refine the innovation to fit the organization,[4] the new practice is more likely to be successfully implemented and sustained. To enhance adoption of the new practice, the EBP team should design the conduct of the pilot to include formal and informal surveys in which the stakeholders on the pilot units can share their opinions and suggestions about the new practice with the EBP team. Team members need to clearly communicate to stakeholders that their input during the pilot will be used when evaluating the need for adapting the new practice. A formal input mechanism could be a simple questionnaire asking specific questions about the practicality of the new practice, as well as open-ended questions asking for the stakeholders' opinions. The informal input mechanism could be verbal inquiry of stakeholders by EBP team members daily during the pilot.

Second, successful adoption of a new practice requires that the stakeholders have a clear understanding of the details of the innovation and how it could affect them, adequate training to use it, and support for fitting it into their work patterns.[4,20] To enhance adoption of the new practice, the EBP team should plan educational strategies to teach stakeholders about the new practice. Educational strategies could include educational sessions, educational materials, and computer-based learning modules. The team should design opportunities for each stakeholder to learn the details of the new practice and expectations for their performance.

Third, stakeholders are more likely to adopt a new practice when proponents of the innovation include local opinion leaders and change champions whose opinions are viewed as credible.[4,6,21–25] Both local opinion leaders and change champions are knowledgeable clinicians whose expertise is valued by other clinicians.[26,27] A change champion tends to take an active role in leading all the steps in an EBP change and to be a role model for the new practice.[28] In some circumstances, a local opinion leader may also function as a change champion. To enhance adoption of the new practice, the EBP team should consider recruiting an opinion leader on each pilot unit to positively promote the adoption of the new practice. Some EBP team members will function as change champions during the pilot. They also should consider recruiting other direct-care nurses as change champions so that there will be a change champion on each shift to promote the adoption of the new practice. The team must provide educational sessions to all change champions first so that they become experienced in the new practice before they act as role models for the practice.

Fourth, audit and feedback about the performance of a new practice has led to successful adoption of the new practice.[5,29–32] To enhance the adoption of the new practice, the EBP team should design a formal mechanism for collecting data about the performance of the new practice during the pilot. A simple approach would be to have the designated EBP team members use the process indicators portion of the project's DCI to collect the performance data. During the early days of the pilot, such data should be collected daily on each opportunity to perform the new practice. Then the EBP team members should provide performance feedback to the responsible stakeholder. This feedback should be delivered in a positive manner to minimize resistance to the new practice by the stakeholder. If the performance data indicate that the stakeholder has performed the new practice as expected, the EBP team member should commend the stakeholder. If the performance data indicate that the stakeholder has not performed the new practice as expected, the EBP team member should remind the responsible stakeholder about performance expectations, inquire about the reasons for not performing the new practice, and troubleshoot any problems. As the pilot progresses and the data indicate that the new practice is being performed somewhat consistently, the EBP team may choose to collect data from a sample of the opportunities to perform the new practice, rather than from 100 percent of such opportunities.

Decide on the time interval for the pilot

When designing the pilot of the new practice, the team must choose the length of time during which the pilot will be run before the postimplementation evaluation is conducted. Six to eight weeks is generally an adequate length of time for staff members to become familiar with the new practice. However, unique organizational characteristics may influence the length of time chosen. For instance, if the pilot is conducted on a small nursing unit with very few staff members, the team may decide to conduct the pilot for only four weeks.

Design the plan for monitoring the fidelity of the pilot

The EBP team cannot assume that the stakeholders will use the new practice automatically once it "goes live." Therefore, the members must design a plan for monitoring the fidelity of the pilot. This means that, after all staff members have received education about the new practice and know the expectations for their performance, designated members of the EBP team or other appointed personnel, such as change champions, will follow up daily on every shift to determine whether the new practice is being performed. The fidelity monitoring plan uses audit and feedback, as described earlier, to provide individualized feedback to each staff member who was responsible for performing the new practice on a specific occasion. The EBP member providing the individualized feedback provides positive reinforcement to the staff members who correctly performed the new practice and positive encouragement to use the new practice to those staff members who did not perform the new practice as expected. The fidelity monitoring plan also incorporates the informal opportunity for the staff members to participate in shaping the new practice, as discussed earlier, by inquiring about opinions regarding how well the new practice is fitting into each staff member's work life and about suggestions for "tweaking" the new practice to make it a better fit. By writing the fidelity monitoring plan, the EBP team can avoid relying on memory.

Design the marketing plan

There is excellent evidence that simply educating health-care providers about a new practice is necessary but not sufficient to promote its adoption.[5] The EBP team should develop a marketing plan to widely disseminate information about the upcoming pilot of the new practice. The team should consider all practical mechanisms for information dissemination that are available within the organization. Developing this plan includes creative thinking about what would appeal to stakeholders, pique their interest, and be difficult to ignore. This is an area where members of organizations are likely to have much experience because marketing plans are used for a vast array of forthcoming changes. Examples of marketing mechanisms include

- Consulting with the organization's marketing director for ideas and for budgetary support, if indicated
- Hosting a round-the-clock "go live" food reception conveniently located on each pilot unit
- Displaying announcement posters on easels in prominent locations that do not obstruct the flow of traffic
- Presenting announcements in monthly staff meetings
- Sending voice mail announcements about the upcoming new practice change to staff members on the pilot units
- Sending e-mail announcements to staff members on the pilot units
- Including an announcement in the unit's monthly newsletter
- Having EBP team members wear large "ask me about … *name of the new practice*" buttons and distributing those buttons to staff members who have completed the education session
- Placing an announcement flyer in each nurse's mailbox
- Attaching an announcement flyer to each nurse's paycheck
- Posting an announcement flyer on toilet doors facing the toilet (an old-time favorite!)
- Displaying posters showing a vertical ruler indicating progressive percent compliance with performance of the new practice, based on the ongoing audit data
- Giving staff name tag lanyards printed with the name of the new practice or a relevant, catchy slogan

The selection of marketing mechanisms will be dependent on the organization's resources and the EBP team members' perceptions of which mechanisms will be effective. Some of the suggestions just listed require existing high technology, while others are low technology. Some represent budget expenditures, while others do not.

Once the pilot is underway, the EBP team should use some of the same marketing mechanisms as periodic reminders to use the new practice. Good evidence indicates that the use of a reminder mechanism enhances adoption of the new practice.[5] Team members must use their judgment about which marketing mechanisms are most effective with their stakeholders and the frequency of the reminders. The goal is to remind, not to harass. By writing the marketing plan, the EBP team can avoid relying on memory.

Assign responsibilities and plan timelines

As the EBP team members are designing the practice change and various components for implementation of the pilot, they will simultaneously begin deciding who will be responsible for the various tasks and planning timelines for the activities of Step 4 and for the pilot activities. There is an obvious sequence for completing the activities of Step 4:

- Define the proposed change.
- Identify the needed resources.
- Design the pilot study.
    — Prepare the new practice documents.
    — Design the materials for monitoring the fidelity of the intervention.
    — Prepare the marketing materials.
    — Design the educational session and educational materials about the new practice.
    — Prepare the change champions for their role.
    — Design the prepilot and postpilot evaluation instruments.
    — Collect the prepilot data and plan the postpilot data collection.

Typically, team members will volunteer for the responsibilities in which they have the most interest, knowledge, and experience. The entire team will participate in defining the proposed change and identifying the needed resources. However, it may be most efficient for smaller subgroups to work simultaneously on the components of designing the pilot study, with some preparing the educational sessions and resources, others designing the marketing plan, and so on. This would be a good time to add a nurse educator from the education department to the team to help with developing the educational sessions and resources for use during the pilot and later. Once drafts of the various components are finished, the entire team should meet to discuss and approve or revise those components.

The EBP team also needs to develop timelines for the activities involved in conducting the pilot. Timing must be decided for these activities:

- Initiation of the marketing plan
- The "go live" date for expecting the staff to begin using the new practice
- Audit and feedback and informal staff opinion surveys in the fidelity monitoring plan
- Formal staff opinion surveys
- Discussion of the progress of the pilot, including ongoing review of the audit results by the EBP team members
- Postpilot data collection
- Analysis of postpilot data and informal and formal staff opinion surveys
- Recommendations regarding adapting, adopting, or rejecting the new practice

The team should strive to be realistic in setting the various timelines, with consideration being given to the typical amount of time required to accomplish group work within the organization. Selection of the timeline for some activities is dependent upon the completion of another activity. For instance, the go live date for using the new practice is dependent upon the marketing plan being fully implemented. Also, collection of the postpilot data is dependent on completion of the pilot phase for the use of the new practice. The audit and feedback and informal staff surveys should start the first day after the go live date but then are ongoing throughout the pilot and end before the postpilot data collection begins.

Obtain Agency Approvals for Pilot

Having completed the design of the new practice and the pilot implementation plan, the team must obtain any necessary agency approvals for proceeding with the pilot. The approvals most likely to be needed are from the unit manager and administrator, the standards and practice committee, and the forms committee, if a new form is being proposed. The necessity of obtaining such approvals is highly dependent on the infrastructure and culture of the organization. If the leadership is centralized, these approvals are more likely to be needed than if the leadership is decentralized. For instance, at WVUH, the leadership is decentralized. Members of the EBP teams include directors and the unit managers; thus, their approval is inherent in the design of the new practice and the implementation plan. This leadership arrangement eliminates the delays inherent in seeking approvals from leadership and relevant committees.

Prepare Pilot Sites

Finally, in Step 4, the EBP team must prepare the sites for the pilot. This requires networking with all levels of unit nurse leaders to recruit their support for conducting the pilot. Preparing the sites also requires conducting the education sessions, distributing the educational materials, and providing access information for any computer-based learning modules. The team must provide all documents and any new forms, equipment, and other materials that the staff members will need if they are to use the new practice. The use of these materials should be well described during the educational sessions and in educational materials. The team must also provide the unit nurse leaders with the names and contact information for the pilot coordinator and the unit's change champions, should issues arise that need troubleshooting. Having designed the practice change, the EBP team moves forward to Step 5 of the EBP model.

Case 6-3 *Planning for the Pilot of the Fabricated CHF Practice Change*

Patients with CHF are admitted to a variety of nursing units. The CHF EBP team decided to conduct the pilot on all of those units to ensure the inclusion of all CHF patients. The majority of the process variables were the responsibility of the two CHF nurse specialists, with only one variable, referral of CHF patients to the nurse specialists, being the direct-care nurses' responsibility. Because of the simplicity of that one activity, the team anticipated minimal resistance by direct-care nurses. The team estimated that a patient sample of 60 would be needed and also estimated that it would be able to recruit 80 patients, to oversample in case of attrition, in four months. Because the team would measure the outcomes for each patient at six months, the pilot would be conducted for ten months. This time interval would allow accumulation of a data set with a minimum of six months of data from each patient. The team acknowledged that this is longer than most pilots, but it was necessary because the team wished to match each patient's initial SCHFI score with the six-month score for comparison.

The specific process and outcome indicators had changed since the team created the CHF DCI in Step 1. For efficiency, the team arranged for Information Technology personnel to work with the two CHF nurse specialists to design an electronic CHF database with prompts for assessment and documentation of the care provided to each patient. Information Technology personnel also created a link to the daily census report with a search query for CHF as the admitting diagnosis. The prompts included:

- Daily generation of new patient records in the CHF database for CHF patients admitted within the past 24 hours
  — This feature notified the CHF nurse specialists of target patients and included a field to document referral by a staff nurse
- Fields for documenting
  — The initial and six-month scores for the SCHFI[17]
  — Initial assessment of patient motivations and barriers to self-care

— Individualized initial and biweekly teaching of CHF self-care
— Biweekly health assessments by telephone
— CHF readmissions

Information Technology personnel developed queries for generating reports on the process and outcome variables. These reports provided information for ongoing monitoring of the effectiveness of the new practice. The creation of the database, with its prompts and query reports, also provided for monitoring the fidelity of the pilot, designing the evaluation instruments, and collecting and analyzing the data.

In consultation with the organization's CHF specialist physician and expert CHF nurse specialists at other organizations, the EBP team decided on an educational strategy for the two new CHF nurse specialists. The strategy included selected readings, online tutorials, shadowing an expert CHF nurse specialist at another organization for two weeks, and an arrangement for telephone consultation with both the organization's CHF specialist physician and an expert CHF nurse specialist at another organization. Educational sessions were also arranged for the two CHF nurse specialists to learn how to use the CHF database.

The team also developed a brief educational session and flyer for introducing the direct-care nurses to their responsibility of referring all CHF patients to the two CHF nurse specialists. The organization's CHF specialist physician advised the team about preparing informational flyers for distribution to the medical staff.

To encourage direct-care nurses to refer CHF patients to the two CHF specialist nurses, the team chose to use audit and feedback for the first month of the pilot. The plan was to have a change champion on every shift of every adult unit conduct the audit and feedback during that month. The team also chose to use e-mail and voice mail to market the new practice. After the first month, the change champions would conduct audit and feedback randomly. They would use e-mail and voice mail if the audit results indicated the need.

The evaluation plan that the team developed consisted of:

- Collecting data from all CHF patients, using the Self-Care of Heart Failure Index,[17] during the period when IT was developing the CHF electronic database, the two CHF nurse specialists and direct-care nurses were attending their respective educational sessions, and the marketing plan was being implemented

- Analysis of the difference among the baseline, the initial (pilot phase) scores, and six-month (postpilot phase) scores for the Self-Care of Heart Failure Index[17]

- Analysis of the cumulative compliance with the expectations to perform:
  — Referral of CHF patients to the nurse specialists by direct-care nurses
  — Initial assessment of patient motivations and barriers to self-care
  — Individualized initial and biweekly teaching of CHF self-care
  — Biweekly telephone health assessments

- Comparison of the cumulative number of CHF readmissions using six months of data for each patient with the number of CHF readmissions for the previous year.

Having planned the pilot, the team obtained approval of the pilot from the chief nurse executive and the chief of the medical staff. Subsequently, the team proceeded with educating participating personnel and disseminating the flyers to physicians, preliminary to starting Step 5 in the EBP model.

REFERENCES

1. Dirksen CD, Ament AJ, Go PM. Diffusions of six surgical endoscopic procedures in the Netherlands: Stimulating and restraining factors. *Health Pol.* 1996;37(2):91–104.
2. Marshall SK. Diffusion of innovations theory and end-user searching. *Library & Information Science Research.* 1990; 6(1):55–69.

3. Meyer M, Johnson D, Ethington C. Contrasting attributes of preventive health innovations. *J Commun*. 1997;47:112–131.

4. Rogers EM. *Diffusion of Innovations*. 4th ed. New York: Free Press; 1995.

5. Greenhalgh T, Robert G, Macfarlane F, et al. Diffusion of innovations in service organizations: Systematic review and recommendations. *Milbank Q*. 2004;82(4):581–629.

6. Meyer AD, Goes JB. Organizational assimilation of innovations: A multi-level contextual analysis. *Acad Manage Rev*. 1988;31:897–923.

7. Denis JL, Hebert Y, Langley A, et al. Explaining diffusion patterns for complex health care innovations. *Health Care Manage Rev*. 2002;27(3):60–73.

8. Grilli R, Lomas J. Evaluating the message: The relationship between compliance rate and the subject of a practice guideline. *Med Care*. 1994;32(3):202–213.

9. Aubert BA, Hamel G. Adoption of smart cards in the medical sector: The Canadian experience. *Soc Sci Med*. 2001;53(7):879–894.

10. Sparks A, Boyer D, Gambrel A, et al. The clinical benefits of the bladder scanner: A research synthesis. *J Nurs Care Qual*. Jul–Sep 2004;19(3):188–192.

11. Gustafson DH, Sainfort F, Eichler M, et al. Developing and testing a model to predict outcomes of organizational change. *Health Serv Res*. 2003;38(2):751–776.

12. St. Clair K, Larrabee JH. Clean vs. sterile gloves: Which to use for postoperative dressing changes? *Outcomes Manage*. 2002;6(1):17–21.

13. Fanning MF. Child Visitation in the Cardiothoracic/Coronary Care Unit. Paper presented at International Nursing Research, the 18th Annual Conference sponsored by the Southern Nursing Research Society; February 19, 2004; Louisville, KY.

14. The Joint Commission. *Comprehensive Accreditation Manual for Hospitals: The Official Handbook*. Oakbrook Terrace, IL: The Joint Commission; 2008.

15. Rumsey DJ. *Statistics for Dummies*. Hoboken, NJ: Wiley; 2003.

16. Gonick L, Smith W. *The Cartoon Guide to Statistics*. New York: HarperPerennial; 1993.

17. Riegel B, Carlson B, Moser DK, et al. Psychometric testing of the self-care of heart failure index. *J Card Fail.* Aug 2004;10(4):350–360.

18. Bennis WG, Benne KD, Chin R (eds.). *The Planning of Change; Readings in the Applied Behavioral Sciences.* New York: Holt Rinehart and Winston; 1964.

19. Ouchi WG. *Theory Z: How American Business Can Meet the Japanese Challenge.* Reading, MA: Addison-Wesley; 1987.

20. Hall GE, Hord SM. *Change in Schools.* Albany, NY: State University of New York Press; 1987.

21. Fitzgerald L, Ferlie E, Wood M, Hawkins C. Interlocking interactions, the diffusion of innovations in health care. *Hum Relat.* 2002;55(12):1429–1449.

22. Locock L, Dopson S, Chambers D, Gabbay J. Understanding the role of opinion leaders in improving clinical effectiveness. *Soc Sci Med.* 2001;53:745–757.

23. Thomson O'Brien MA, Oxman AD, Haynes RB, et al. Local opinion leaders: Effects on professional practice and health care outcomes. *The Cochrane Library.* 2004;4:4.

24. Backer TE, Rogers EM. Diffusion of innovations theory and work-site AIDS programs. *J Community Health.* Jan–Mar 1998;3(1):17–28.

25. Markham SK. A longitudinal examination of how champions influence others to support their projects. *J Product Innovation Manag.* 1998;15(6):490–504.

26. Craig JV, Smyth RL. *The Evidence-Based Practice Manual for Nurses.* 2nd ed. Edinburgh, NY: Churchill Livingstone; 2007.

27. Oxman AD, Thomson MA, Davis DA, Haynes RB. No magic bullets: A systematic review of 102 trials of interventions to improve professional practice. *Can Med Assoc J.* Nov 15 1995;153(10):1423–1431.

28. Ardery G, Herr K, Hannon BJ, Titler MG. Lack of opioid administration in older hip fracture patients (CE). *Geriatr Nurs.* Nov–Dec 2003;24(6):353–360.

29. Titler MG. Translation science: Quality, methods and issues. *Community Nurs Res.* 2004;37:15, 17–34.

30. Green PL. Improving clinical effectiveness in an integrated care delivery system. *J Healthc Qual.* Nov–Dec 1998;20(6):4–8; quiz 9, 48.
31. Grimshaw JM, Thomas RE, MacLennan G, et al. Effectiveness and efficiency of guideline dissemination and implementation strategies. *Health Technol Assess.* Feb 2004;8(6):iii–iv, 1–72.
32. Jamtvedt G, Young JM, Kristoffersen DT, et al. Audit and feedback: Effects on professional practice and health care outcomes. *Cochrane Database Syst Rev: Rev.* 2006(Issue 2).

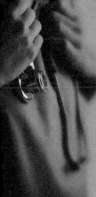

Chapter 7

STEP 5: IMPLEMENT AND EVALUATE CHANGE IN PRACTICE

■ **IMPLEMENT THE PILOT STUDY**

—Initiate Use of the Practice Change at the Designated Time
—Provide Follow-Up Reinforcement of the Practice Change
—Obtain Feedback from Stakeholders

■ **EVALUATE PROCESSES, OUTCOMES, AND COSTS**

—Obtain an Adequate Sample Size
—Verify the Accuracy of the Data
—Conduct Data Analysis

■ **DEVELOP CONCLUSIONS AND RECOMMENDATIONS**

—Discuss Evaluation Summaries
—Decide to Adapt, Adopt, or Reject the Practice Change

In this step, the evidence-based practice (EBP) team will implement the pilot study of the new practice and evaluate the processes, outcomes, and costs. Then they will develop conclusions and recommendations.

IMPLEMENT THE PILOT STUDY

Initiate Use of the Practice Change at the Designated Time

Having prepared the pilot sites and educated the stakeholders about the new practice, the EBP team initiates the pilot study of the new practice at the designated time. It is important for the pilot coordinator, local opinion leaders, and change champions to be available to the stakeholders, especially the first day and first week of the pilot. Responding promptly to stakeholders who have questions or concerns can minimize their frustration with performing the new practice. Such interactions also allow the pilot coordinator and the EBP team members to troubleshoot any unanticipated problems early in the pilot.

Provide Follow-Up Reinforcement of the Practice Change

As planned in Step 4, the EBP team will conduct audit and feedback. The responsible change champions will begin identifying occasions when the new practice should have been performed within the first 24 hours after it "goes live." The change champions will use the process indicators section of the data collection instrument (DCI) to evaluate whether or not the processes of the new practice were performed on each occasion when they should have been. The change champions will also identify the staff member who was responsible for performing the new practice on each occasion. Using the information collected, the change champions will discuss the information collected with the responsible staff member, commending the staff member for processes that were performed correctly and clarifying expectations about processes that were not performed correctly. As mentioned in Step 4, such conversations should be handled in a positive manner, rather than in a punitive manner, to minimize resistance to the new practice.

Reinforcement of the new practice is also achieved by implementing the ongoing marketing plan developed in Step 4. The team will use the marketing mechanisms and timing selected. As the pilot progresses, the team and the change champions should discuss how the stakeholders are reacting to the marketing mechanisms and their timing. That information may suggest the need for some adjustments in the ongoing marketing plan. For instance, if the plan included a poster on an easel and stakeholders comment that the easel is obstructing the flow of traffic, the team could elicit suggestions for a better location. If no good location can be identified, the team should remove the poster and the easel.

Obtain Feedback from Stakeholders

The EBP team will follow through with the informal and formal input mechanisms selected in Step 4. The informal mechanism of obtaining feedback from stakeholders occurs simultaneously with audit and feedback. It should also include asking nurse leaders on each pilot unit for their feedback on how the pilot is progressing and any concerns that they have about the new practice. If other disciplines are stakeholders of the new practice, the team should ask for their feedback also. As informal feedback data are obtained, the EBP team member or change champion obtaining them writes notes about the comments. These are shared with the team and the change champions in periodic pilot project meetings, to keep everyone informed as the pilot progresses. At the conclusion of the pilot, the responsible team member will summarize all the informal feedback.

At the planned time, the team will distribute to stakeholders the simple questionnaire designed in Step 4 as the formal input mechanism. A simple strategy for collecting the completed questionnaires is to ask stakeholders to deposit them in a sealed collection box. The team will tally the responses on the completed questionnaires, for use after the pilot phase.

EVALUATE PROCESSES, OUTCOMES, AND COSTS

When the pilot phase has ended, the EBP team will conduct the postpilot evaluation. This includes obtaining an adequate sample size, verifying the accuracy of the data, conducting data analysis, and interpreting the results.

Obtain an Adequate Sample Size

The data collectors will collect process, outcome, and cost data according to the evaluation plan developed in Step 4. That work continues until the needed sample size is obtained. The estimate of the length of time that would be required to obtain the needed sample size may or may not have been accurate. Factors that may influence the length of time required to obtain the needed sample size include a change in the volume of appropriate patients, variances in the length of time required to collect the data, and staffing needs that unexpectedly prevent the data collectors from being out of staffing to collect data.

Verify the Accuracy of the Data

Once the data collection has been completed, the EBP team member responsible for analysis will examine the data for accuracy. This is done by examining each DCI for data-entry errors. For example, in the excerpt from the DCI in Figure 3-6 shown here, the percent compliance with criterion 3 is wrong:

Chart Review Form: Chronic Heart Failure Nursing Care

ANSWER CODE:	1 = YES	0 = NO	ND = Not Documented	NA = Not Applicable

3. (a) How many times *should* nurse have performed every 8-hour assessment?	7
(b) How many times did nurse *actually* perform every 8-hour assessment?	10
% compliance	80

7. RN taught patient self-care needed after discharge for	
(a) Medicines	1
(b) Weight management (fluid restrictions)	0
(c) Signs and symptoms needing physician attention	2

In addition, in the excerpt from the DCI in Figure 3-6, the answer to criterion 7c is wrong because the possible answers for this criterion are 1 = yes, 0 = no, ND = not documented, and NA = not applicable. The data analyst corrects any data-entry errors that are identified. When the error is a calculation error, the data analyst will recalculate to obtain the correct number. When the error is not a calculation error, such as in the example using criterion 7, the data collector must try to recall the correct answer. Alternatively, if the source of data is a document, such as the medical record, the data collector should examine that document again and provide the data analyst with the corrected DCI.

Conduct Data Analysis

Depending on how the DCI was designed, the nature of the criteria, and the sample size, the data analysis may consist of tallying results by hand. If the data were entered into an Excel spreadsheet, the data analyst can use the formula menu to calculate the results. The use of an electronic spreadsheet is especially efficient when the sample size is large. Also, there are less likely to be calculation errors when an electronic spreadsheet is used, as long as no errors were made when entering data from the DCI forms. To confirm that there are no data-entry errors, the data analyst should compare the data on the DCI with the data in the spreadsheet. In addition, the data analyst can calculate frequencies and examine them for any wrong response codes, as in the example using criterion 7c. For a criterion such as number 3 in the DCI in Figure 3-6, with a percent as an answer, the mean and standard deviation can be calculated for the sample. For a criterion such as number 7 in the DCI in Figure 3-6, with a simple yes/no response, frequency and percent can be calculated for the sample. When the pilot occurred on more than one unit, the data analyst can also calculate results by unit if there is a data field for "unit" for each row of data. As described in Step 1, the data analyst can use Excel to generate histograms displaying results for each criterion at one time or multiple times. Also, Excel can generate histograms comparing units on the process and outcome indicators. The data analyst prepares a summary of the analysis and results.

DEVELOP CONCLUSIONS AND RECOMMENDATIONS

Discuss Evaluation Summaries

The EBP team uses the analysis and results summary to discuss and interpret the results. The results will indicate the extent to which the desired patient outcomes are being achieved and the extent to which the processes of the new practice are being performed during the postpilot period. If an opportunity for improvement exists, this information should be used to identify the corrective actions that are needed. Sometimes the marketing plan and the audit and feedback will not be robust enough to persuade stakeholders to perform the new practice.

If the team comes to that conclusion, then more robust marketing and audit and feedback should be developed. Otherwise, the team should consider additional strategies demonstrated to be effective in promoting the adoption of a new practice. One example is reminders in the form of prompts programmed into the electronic medical record system.

If cost data were collected and analyzed, the team will discuss and interpret those results also. Such data provide useful information for judging the budgetary feasibility of the practice change within the organization. Even if the evidence base reviewed in Step 3 included evidence of the cost-effectiveness of a new practice, that conclusion may not hold true in a particular organization because organizational characteristics vary widely.

Although the EBP team and change champions discussed the informal feedback from stakeholders as the pilot progressed, the team will now discuss that feedback together with the formal feedback, using the summaries of those data. As they discuss the feedback, team members compare and contrast the comments with their own assessment of the new practice and how well the pilot progressed. Negative themes that are common warrant consideration because they suggest that resistance to performing the new practice could be reduced if the relevant aspect of the new practice were modified. For instance, suppose that one process in a new practice was to document the practice on a new form that required the entry of data that are already required on another documentation form. If a common theme in the feedback is objection to using the new form, and if the audit data during the pilot and the evaluation of process data indicate that the form was being used less than 50 percent of the time, the team should consider whether an existing form could be used to document the performance of the new practice.

Decide to Adapt, Adopt, or Reject the Practice Change

Following critical analysis of all the data summaries, the EBP team decides whether to adapt, adopt, or reject the new practice. The most common decision is to adapt the new practice slightly to better fit the organization. Despite stakeholder representation on the EBP team, it is possible that the new practice is not a perfect fit with the organization when it is piloted. If the EBP team has followed the EBP model and made correct judgments about the strength of the evidence, it is unlikely that it will reach the end of Step 5 and decide to reject the new practice.

When adapting the description of the new practice based on the need identified in the evaluation data, the team must attempt to keep the processes of the new practice consistent with those supported in the evidence base. The adaptation of documentation discussed in the previous section does not contradict the evidence base, as the base did not include specifics about how to document the new practice.

 CASE 7-1 *Implementing and Evaluating the New Practice for the Fabricated Chronic Heart Failure (CHF) EBP Project*

The pilot of the new practice was initiated after the CHF nurse specialists and the direct-care nurses had completed their respective educational sessions and the initial marketing plan had been implemented. The change champions initiated audit and feedback on every shift of every adult unit within 24 hours of going live. This activity continued daily for the first month and then was scaled back to one day a week for the rest of the pilot. When the audit results warranted, the change champions used e-mail and voice mail as a reminder to make referrals to the two CHF nurse specialists.

Meanwhile, the two CHF nurse specialists performed the responsibilities of their role, providing care to CHF patients while they were hospitalized and via telephone after hospital discharge. They generated weekly reports of the process indicators of care and CHF readmissions. Because the electronic database generated a record in the database for CHF patients admitted within the past 24 hours, the two CHF nurse specialists could identify when a direct-care nurse failed to make a referral. The CHF nurse specialists notified the appropriate change champion to follow up with the direct-care nurse, as a reminder. After the patient had been followed for six months, the CHF nurse specialists collected the six-month Self-Care of Heart Failure Index (SCHFI) data and entered them into the electronic database.

By the end of the pilot, the EBP team had six-month data for 56 patients; therefore, the pilot phase was extended by two weeks to obtain the needed sample of 60 CHF patients. The CHF electronic database was used to calculate the cumulative compliance with the expectations to perform

- Referral of CHF patients to the nurse specialists by direct-care nurses
- Initial assessment of patient motivations and barriers to self-care
- Individualized initial and biweekly teaching of CHF self-care
- Biweekly telephone health assessments

Because of the nature of the analyses needed, an employee in Support Services conducted these analyses:

- Analysis of the difference among the baseline, the initial (pilot phase), and the six-month (postpilot) scores for the SCHFI[1]
- Comparison of the cumulative number of CHF readmissions for each patient with the number of CHF readmissions for 10 months preceding the pilot

The results of the analyses were:

Referral of CHF patients to the nurse specialists by direct-care nurses	85%
Initial assessment of patient motivations and barriers to self-care	100%
Individualized initial teaching of CHF self-care	100%
Individualized biweekly teaching of CHF self-care	80%
Biweekly telephone health assessments	80%

Analysis of the differences among the baseline, the initial pilot phase, and the six-month postpilot phase scores for the SCHFI[1] indicated that the baseline and the initial pilot phase scores did not differ statistically. However, the mean SCHFI score at six months was 8 percent higher than the initial SCHIFI score, indicating improvement in reported self-care. The cumulative number of CHF readmissions for each patient in the pilot was 8 percent lower than the number of CHF readmissions for 10 months prior to the pilot, suggesting that the new practice was effective. Still, the goal had been to improve both of those outcomes by 10 percent.

The EBP team discussed the evaluation results and concluded that, overall, the new practice was effective, although there remained opportunity for improvement in the outcomes and in three of the processes of care. The team recommended continuation of the new practice with adaptations to address those three processes. First, because only 85 percent of patients with CHF were referred to the nurse specialists by direct-care nurses, the team recommended that Information Technology add a prompt for direct-care nurses to make the referral when a patient with CHF is admitted. The two CHF nurse specialists met the expectations of performing individualized biweekly teaching of CHF self-care and biweekly telephone health assessments only 80 percent of the time. Reasons included their being unable to reach some patients by telephone during a two-week period and finding that some patients did not have a telephone. The team recommended adding toll-free numbers so that CHF patients could make calls to the CHF nurse specialists. For patients without a telephone, the CHF nurse specialists would mail postcards to patients with a reminder that it was time for follow-up and encouraging them to call the toll-free number when they could get access to a telephone. For patients with telephones whom the nurses have difficulty reaching in a two-week period, the nurses would mail a similar reminder card asking the patients to call one of the nurses when they had time.

The EBP members observed that some CHF patients were not receiving the care available from the CHF nurse specialists because they were not being coded as having CHF until after discharge. Therefore, the team recommended that it work on resolving that issue as its next project and further adapt the practice after feasible solutions are identified. The team summarized the project, results, and recommendations in a one-page bulleted "talking points" document for use in Step 6. Having decided on specific adaptations to the new practice, the team is ready to initiate Step 6 in the EBP change model.

REFERENCE

1. Riegel B, Carlson B, Moser DK, et al. Psychometric testing of the self-care of heart failure index. J Card Fail. Aug 2004;10(4): 350–360.

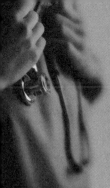

STEP 6: INTEGRATE AND MAINTAIN CHANGE IN PRACTICE

- **COMMUNICATE THE RECOMMENDED CHANGE TO STAKEHOLDERS**
  — Present Staff In-Service Education on Change in Practice
- **INTEGRATE INTO STANDARDS OF PRACTICE**
- **MONITOR THE PROCESS AND OUTCOMES PERIODICALLY**
- **CELEBRATE AND DISSEMINATE THE RESULTS OF THE PROJECT**

In this step, the evidence-based practice (EBP) team will communicate the recommended practice change to stakeholders and integrate it into standards of practice. Then, the EBP team will make plans for ongoing monitoring of the process and outcome indicators.

COMMUNICATE THE RECOMMENDED CHANGE TO STAKEHOLDERS

Present Staff In-Service Education on Change in Practice

Having decided either to adopt the practice change or to adapt it, the EBP team next communicates the recommendations to all stakeholders. Stakeholders include nurse leaders, physician leaders, all personnel who will be expected to perform the new practice, physicians whose patients will receive care using the new practice, and relevant patients. Other stakeholders depend on the nature of the new practice and could include other disciplines, such as pharmacists, respiratory therapists, dieticians, and social workers.

First, the EBP team members present their recommendations to nurse leaders and appropriate physician leaders, using the "talking points" document developed in Step 5 to obtain final approval. If those leaders agree that the evaluation summary supports adopting or adapting the new practice, they are very likely to approve it. If the evaluation summary also indicates that the benefits associated with the new practice justify the costs, the leaders are very likely to approve it. However, if the costs seem high relative to the benefits, the leaders may either disapprove the change or ask the EBP team to consider alternatives with lower costs.

Second, recommendations about the new practice must be communicated to all personnel who will be expected to perform it. If all units for which the new practice is relevant participated in the pilot, the communication will be limited to the evaluation results and any recommendations for adapting any of the processes of care. If not all units for which the new practice is relevant participated in the pilot, the communication will consist of the evaluation results, the in-service education presented to stakeholders on pilot units prior to the pilot, and any adaptation of processes. Based on the evaluation results and their observations during the pilot, the EBP team members decide whether any changes in the in-service education are needed before scheduling educational sessions.

Because of staff turnover, plans must be made to include in-service education covering the new practice in the orientation of new employees. The EBP team collaborates with a member of the education department to initiate this integration. Subsequently, a member of the education department will be responsible for consistently including this in-service education in all future orientations, until such time as further adaptations in the practice are made.

Third, the EBP team must communicate with physicians whose patients will receive care using the new practice. The team should reexamine the materials and strategies used to introduce the new practice to physicians prior to the pilot. If there were adaptations in any processes of the practice, the team should update those materials and strategies. If the new practice is being adopted without adaptations, the original materials and strategies can be used in conjunction with the talking points document to inform physicians about the evaluation results and the decision to make the new practice a standard of care.

Fourth, the EBP team must decide how to communicate the recommendations to patients and their families so that they know what to expect with their care. The team may decide that a brief flyer would be effective for some patients. Verbal explanations accompanying the flyer would be helpful for patients who cannot read, because of either illiteracy, lack of access to their eyeglasses, or their current physical status. For example, if a patient is unconscious or has cognitive impairment, family members should be informed about what to expect. These communications would be delivered by direct-care nurses. The team would need to prepare the flyer and any instructions the direct-care nurses would need.

Fifth, the EBP team must decide how to communicate the recommendations to stakeholders other than those who are expected to perform the new practice and physicians. It would be most efficient if the same materials and strategies used when communicating with those who are expected to perform the new practice or physicians could be used.

INTEGRATE INTO STANDARDS OF PRACTICE

In Step 4, the EBP team described the processes of the new practice in a document such as a procedure, policy, care map, or guideline, based on the preference of nurse leaders. Such documents are considered standards of care. If the new practice is being adopted without adaptations, the original document does not need to be revised. If the new practice is being adopted with process adaptations, the EBP team will edit the document describing the new practice to reflect those process adaptations. Depending on the organizational structure, the EBP team may need to obtain final approval of the new standard of care by the standards and practice committee.

If the new practice had required a new documentation form and the new practice is being adopted with process adaptations, the EBP team will edit the form to address the adapted processes. Depending on the organizational structure, the EBP may need to obtain final approval of the new form from the forms committee.

 CASE 8-1 *Integrating and Maintaining the New Practice for the Fabricated Chronic Heart Failure (CHF) EBP Project*

Members of the EBP team met with nurse leaders and relevant physician leaders, using the talking points document developed in Step 5. The team's recommendations were approved, so the team proceeded to communicate the adapted new practice to the remaining stakeholders. All relevant units had participated in the pilot; therefore, the communication to direct-care nurses included distributing the talking points document via e-mail, voice mail, and individual mailboxes on the units. Members of the team also attended monthly unit meetings to discuss the new practice and answer questions about it. The team also distributed the talking points document to physicians who treat patients with CHF. Patients who were currently in the CHF database received a letter informing them to expect mailed reminder cards about follow-up care if they did not have a telephone or if they could not be reached after four attempted calls during a two-week period.

The policy describing the new practice that was developed during Step 4 was edited to reflect the adaptations in the three processes (Case 7-1). Then, the team discussed the revised policy and the talking points document with the standards and practice committee, which approved the revised policy. Changes pertaining to the three adapted processes were also made in the CHF database by an Information Technology (IT) technician. An IT technician also programmed a prompt in the electronic medical record to alert direct-care nurse when a patient was admitted with a diagnosis of CHF. Finally, the team planned to conduct ongoing monitoring of process and outcome indicators one year from the date of the postpilot data collection period.

MONITOR THE PROCESS AND OUTCOMES PERIODICALLY

When EBP team members arrive at this last activity in Step 6, it is very tempting to consider the project completed and to give little or no attention to ongoing monitoring of the processes and outcomes of the practice. It is quite important for the team to avoid this temptation because, as W. Edwards Deming said: "In God we trust, all others must bring data." Without periodic data collection and analysis using the same process and outcome indicators that were used for the pre/postpilot data analysis, there will be no evidence that the new practice is still being performed correctly and when it should be. There can only be perceptions of whether or not this is so—not the best evidence. Also, without ongoing monitoring, there would be no evidence about the outcomes, only perceptions.

Many EBP teams are a permanent part of the organizational structure, while others are ad hoc. In either case, the EBP team should plan for ongoing monitoring. The intervals between data collection periods may depend, in part, on the level of compliance with the process and outcome indicators in previous data collection periods. In the past, the Joint Commission on Accreditation of Healthcare Organisations introduced the concept of "threshold," meaning a specified percent compliance with a quality indicator. Currently, the Joint Commission requires corrective action when percent compliance with a quality indicator is below the acceptable threshold of 90 to 100 percent compliance. The EBP team should use a desired threshold to decide when corrective action is needed and how frequently monitoring should occur. Depending on the risks to the patient of failing to perform processes correctly or failing to achieve the outcome, the threshold should be set higher than 90 percent. For instance, if the outcome is "no wrong site surgeries," the threshold should be 100 percent. For this outcome indicator, the team would continuously monitor for any occurrence of wrong site surgery. Should one occur, it is considered a sentinel event, and the team must investigate preceding actions that could have caused it and implement corrective action.

If compliance with the process and outcome indicators at previous data collection periods was at what the team considered to be an acceptable threshold, then monitoring once a year should be adequate to inform the team about how well the direct-care nurses are performing the practice. However, if compliance with the process and outcome indicators at previous data collection periods was below what the team considered to be an acceptable threshold, then corrective action should be taken between the data collection periods, and monitoring should occur more frequently, perhaps at three months or six months after the last corrective action. The EBP team can base the decision on how many years to do ongoing monitoring of a practice on the same logic: compliance with the process and outcome indicators at previous data collection periods.

Corrective actions should be focused on the process or outcome indicators that were below the threshold. Talking with some of the stakeholders responsible for performing the new practice could provide insights into the reasons that performance expectations are not being met at the threshold level. This information could be used to decide on corrective action. It may be adequate to give stakeholders feedback on the audit results and reminders about performance expectations. In some instances, knowledge about why the indicator results are below the threshold may lead to "tweaking" of a process that is part of the practice. Suppose that one process in a practice involving bladder scanner use was for the direct-care nurse to obtain a physician's order before each use of the bladder scanner. Further suppose that some nurses said that more time was required to do that than was required to perform an intermittent catheterization. As a result, they were not using the bladder scanner as expected. In such an instance, the EBP team should consider deleting the process requiring nurses to obtain a physician's order. Such an order is not needed because using the bladder scanner is a noninvasive procedure.

To provide structure to ongoing monitoring, the team should consider developing or adopting an annual calendar template. An example of an annual calendar template is given in Figure 8-1, and an example of a completed annual calendar is given in Figure 8-2. When setting tentative deadlines, the team should consider avoiding times of the year that are busier than usual, such as

- Influx of newly graduated nurses
- Annual turnover of medical residents in academic medical centers
- Vacations and holidays

The deadlines should be considered tentative because a variety of factors can influence the amount of time that team members have to work on the project, requiring them to adjust deadlines. Examples of these factors include

- Announced and unannounced accreditation and certification survey visits
- Staffing issues
- Attrition of a team member

Completion Deadlines for 200x Name of Team's Projects

Topic(s)	Jan	Feb	Mar	Apr	May	June	Jul	Aug	Sep	Oct	Nov	Dec

NOTE: Insert in month cell the appropriate code below to indicate targeted completion dates.

- **Step 3** means finishing the synthesis of reviewed literature and deciding if there is sufficient evidence to justify a practice change.
- **Step 6** means completion of postimplementation evaluation of the pilot of the practice change and implementing mechanisms to maintain the practice change over time.
- **QI** means completion of annual follow-up quality improvement monitoring after practice change.

Figure 8-1 Annual calendar template for all of one team's projects planned for a year.

Annual Calendar for 200x   Medical/Surgical Unit EBP Team

Topic(s)	Jan	Feb	Mar	Apr	May	June	Jul	Aug	Sep	Oct	Nov	Dec
Treating intravenous-associated extravasations					Step 3						Step 6	
Managing central line	QI											
Preventing urinary tract infection in patients with indwelling catheters			QI						QI			

NOTE: Insert in month cell the appropriate code below to indicate targeted completion dates.

- **Step 3** means finishing the synthesis of reviewed literature and deciding if there is sufficient evidence to justify a practice change.
- **Step 6** means completion of postimplementation evaluation of the pilot of the practice change and implementing mechanisms to maintain the practice change over time.
- **QI** means completion of annual follow-up quality improvement monitoring after practice change.

Figure 8-2   Example of completed annual calendar.

• Personal issues
  — Illness or family illness
  — Death in the family

For ad hoc teams, the calendar will display only the projected month for the next data collection period. For standing teams, the calendar will display the timing of conducting the new project for the year and the annual, or more frequent, data collection for completed EBP projects. For these teams, the members should consider having a subgroup of the team conduct the annual data collection for the completed projects, so that the rest of the team can focus on the next EBP project. Alternatively, the team could consider recruiting nonteam stakeholders to conduct the annual data collection. This has been an effective strategy in quality improvement because it reinforces for the direct-care nurses who are collecting the data, the importance of correctly performing the practice and correctly documenting performance.

The results of ongoing monitoring may trigger the implementation of corrective actions, as discussed earlier. It also may trigger ideas for new EBP projects. Suppose, for instance, that while collecting observation data about the proper positioning and anchoring of intravenous catheters, EBP team members observe a number of patients with large, painful extravasations from previous intravenous catheters. This observation could lead the team to start a new EBP project focused on the best evidence for treating intravenous-associated extravasations.

CELEBRATE AND DISSEMINATE THE RESULTS OF THE PROJECT

Having completed the six steps of the model for EBP change on their topic, team members should celebrate their successful EBP change and their continued professional learning.

Celebrations will be influenced by the team's imagination, budget, and organization policies. Examples include:

- Team members having a pizza party at one of their scheduled meeting times
- Team members going to lunch together Dutch treat
- Team members organizing an ice cream social for all shifts on all units that participated in the pilot

After celebrating the success of one EBP project and while beginning Step 1 of another project, the team should consider disseminating information about its project organizationwide and outside the organization. Disseminating information organizationwide could include the following:

- Writing a description of the project and the results for the nursing division's newsletter
- Posting a description of the project on the nursing division's research web site
- Preparing a poster for display at the nursing division's annual research day

Disseminating information outside the organization could include

- Writing a description of the project and the results for submission to a clinical journal
- Submitting an abstract for presentation at a local, regional, or national conference

Disseminating information is potentially useful to others who may wish to replicate the project or pilot the recommended new practice in their own setting. For many nurses, writing for publication and presenting at conferences are new learning experiences that further build their professional knowledge and skills. Not all EBP team members will be interested in undertaking these learning experiences. For those who are, seeing their article in print and interacting with other conference attendees can be very rewarding. Whether or not a team member participated in disseminating information outside the organization, the successful completion of an EBP change can be sufficiently rewarding to motivate participation in the next EBP project. Furthermore, the motivation and enthusiasm of even one team member can encourage others to become members of the EBP team.

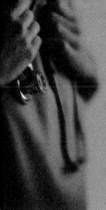

GLOSSARY

Adverse outcome. A patient health-care outcome that causes or has the potential to cause increased morbidity or mortality. Health-care providers strive to prevent adverse outcomes.

Audit and feedback. A strategy for promoting the adoption of an innovation by health-care providers. It consists of preparing a summary of a provider's or a group of providers' performance on a standard of practice. The summary and any recommendations for improvement are shared with the providers.

Benchmarking. The comparison of internal data with either internal data collected at an earlier time or external data.

Brainstorming. A structured or unstructured teamwork tool for idea generation when selecting the clinical problem that is to be the focus of an evidence-based practice project.

Change champion. A knowledgeable clinician whose expertise is valued by other clinicians. The use of change champions is a strategy for promoting the adoption of an innovation by health-care providers. A change champion takes an active role in leading all steps in EBP change and acts as a role model for the new practice.

Clinical practice guideline (CPG). A document that presents recommendations for practice based on systematic reviews of the available evidence.

Confirmability. A trustworthiness criterion that is the qualitative equivalent of objectivity in quantitative research. It pertains to whether the findings reflect the participants' experience and not just the researcher's. To meet this criterion, the report of the qualitative study must provide a sufficiently detailed description of the researcher's own preconceptions and how they influenced decisions throughout the research study.

Control group. A group of study participants in an experiment who do not receive the intervention. This group receives usual care, a placebo, or an alternative intervention.

Credibility. A trustworthiness criterion that is the qualitative equivalent of internal validity in quantitative research. When critically appraising the credibility of a qualitative research study, one seeks to answer this question: do the findings reflect reality? Credibility depends on many aspects of the study, including how well-qualified the researcher was to conduct the study; the extent to which the researcher used an established research tradition; whether or not the sampling plan was appropriate to answer the research question; whether or not the researcher performed "member checks," sharing results with and obtaining feedback from some of the participants; and how in-depth the description of the phenomenon, model of social processes, or culture is.

Critical appraisal. Systematically analyzing research to evaluate its validity, results, and relevance prior to using it to change practice.

Critical appraisal topic (CAT). A structured abstract of a medical journal article prepared by a reviewer of the article.

Data, continuous. Quantitative values that occur in an infinite or unlimited range. Continuous data are produced by interval scales, which assign a number to represent ordered categories of a characteristic for which the intervals between the numbers are equal; however, the zero point is arbitrary, and therefore an interval scale cannot provide information about the exact magnitude of the differences between points on the scale. Temperature has an arbitrary zero, for example.

Data, discrete. Qualitative values that occur in a finite or limited range. Discrete data are produced by nominal scales, which assign a number to represent characteristics of people or things. The assigned numbers for the responses have qualitative, not quantitative, value.

Data, ordinal. Values produced by scales that assign a number to represent categories of a characteristic that are arranged in a meaningful order, such as from low to high.

Data, ratio. Values produced by scales that assign a number to represent meaningfully ordered categories of a characteristic for which the intervals between the numbers are equal and the scale has a true zero. Age has a true zero, for example.

Dependability. A trustworthiness criterion that pertains to whether or not a qualitative study could be replicated by another researcher. To meet this criterion, the report of the qualitative study must provide a sufficiently detailed description of the research design, the procedures used in collecting and analyzing the data, and critical analysis of the research methodology as it was implemented.

Educational sessions or meetings. A strategy for promoting the adoption of an innovation by health-care providers. The use of educational sessions or meetings involves presenting and discussing best practice evidence with health-care providers and encouraging their use of the information in practice.

Effect size. The strength of the relationship between variables; it can vary from very small to large. The power to detect the effect of an intervention is dependent on how large the effect size is and the number of participants. The smaller the effect size to be detected, the larger the sample needed.

Evidence-based practice (EBP). Clinical decision making based on the simultaneous use of the best evidence, clinical expertise, and patients' values.

Experimental group. The group that receives the intervention in an experimental study.

Expert committee reports. Consensus statements that are based primarily on the clinical expertise of the committee members, but may also be based on scientific evidence.

Hierarchy of evidence. A list of evidence in descending order of strength of the evidence, based on the rigor of research and other evidence.

Indicator. A rate-based statement designed to measure evidence of meeting a standard of practice. It may be referred to as a quality indicator. A process indicator measures an action specified by a standard of practice, and an outcome indicator measures a desired consequence of meeting a standard of practice.

Instrument reliability. The consistency with which an instrument measures the variable or underlying concept.

Instrument validity. The degree to which an instrument measures the intended concept.

Internal consistency reliability. A statistical calculation of the homogeneity of the items in an instrument and the subscales within an instrument. Homogeneity of the items or subscales indicates that they are measuring the same concept. Internal consistency reliability is often presented in research reports as a Cronbach alpha (α), together with the significance of the correlations as a probability or p-value ($p = n$, where n = the number value).

Mean. The sum of all observations or scores for a measured variable divided by the number of observations or participants.

Meta-analysis. A type of systematic review that includes the statistical combination of at least two studies to produce a single estimate of the effect of an intervention on an outcome.

Multivoting. A structured teamwork tool for voting on nominated topics in order to choose one as the focus of an evidence-based practice project.

Ongoing monitoring. The periodic measurement and evaluation of process and outcome indicators of quality. Cost of care indicators may also be monitored and evaluated periodically. Ongoing monitoring allows tracking and trending of performance and identification of opportunities for further systems improvement.

Opinion leaders. Knowledgeable clinicians whose expertise and opinions are valued by other clinicians. The use of opinion leaders is a strategy for promoting the adoption of an innovation by health-care providers.

Power. The ability of a research design to identify relationships among measured variables.

Quality improvement (QI). A systematic approach to monitoring and improving systems to achieve better outcomes.

Random assignment. The assignment of study participants in an experiment to the experimental group or the control group by chance, such as using a table of random numbers. Random assignment helps control for confounding or extraneous variables, enhancing the rigor of the experiment.

Research. Scientifically rigorous, systematic inquiry to build a knowledge base.

Research design. The plan describing all aspects of the study, including the data to be collected, data collection instruments, the data collection plan, the intervention (when the study is an experiment), strategies to assure consistency in implementing the intervention, and strategies for controlling for confounding or extraneous variables.

Research, qualitative. The study of human phenomena using holistic methodologies that incorporate contextual influences.

Research, quantitative. Research that describes a concept in depth, presents data about the incidence of a health problem or complication, identifies associations among variables, examines differences between groups or times, identifies predictors of an outcome, or evaluates the effectiveness of an intervention.

Research reports. Written reports describing original research, its findings, and recommendations for practice, if any.

Research utilization (RU). The deliberate, systematic use of research to improve clinical practice and health-care outcomes.

Sentinel event. An adverse event with such dire consequences that each one must be scrutinized for causes to prevent future occurrences.

Stakeholders. Persons who have a stake in the outcome of a health-care practice. Stakeholders include patients and their families, health-care providers, health-care system leaders, and other health system employees.

Standard deviation. A measure of the variation of observations or scores from a variable's mean.

Standards of practice. Statements describing the expected level of health-care practice or performance that are used to evaluate the quality of practice.

Statistical quality control. Activities to identify variability in the quality of products or services through ongoing measurement and system changes to improve work processes as a means of improving products or outcomes of care.

Statistical significance. A statistically calculated measure of the significance of effect size or a relationship. Significance is reported as a probability or p-value. The traditional significance level used in most studies is $p < .05$. A $p < .05$ means that only 5 times out of 100 would an effect or relationship be detected by *chance* instead of because a true effect or relationship exists.

Synthesis. A summary of the current state of knowledge about the topic that was the focus of a literature review. This summary is the state of the science of the reviewed knowledge base.

Systematic review. A critical analysis, using a rigorous methodology, of original research identified by a comprehensive search of the literature.

Transferability. A trustworthiness criterion that considers the extent to which the findings of a qualitative study can be applicable in other settings. Because the findings of a qualitative study are highly dependent upon the context in which the study is conducted, the research report must have a full description of the contextual factors that influenced the findings for readers to judge the potential transferability of the findings to their own setting.

Trustworthiness. A characteristic referring to the rigor of a qualitative study. One set of criteria for evaluating trustworthiness consists of credibility, dependability, confirmability, and transferability.

Validity, external. The applicability of study findings to other settings and populations beyond the site of the study; also known as generalizability. It is largely dependent on the characteristics of the study's sample and how representative the participants are of the general population.

Validity, internal. The extent to which an inference can be made that the independent variable, such as the intervention, influences the dependent variable.

Variable, dependent or outcome. A variable that the researcher aims to identify predictors for or to influence with an intervention.

Variable, extraneous or confounding. A variable other than the independent variable that can influence the dependent variable or the independent variable, confounding the interpretation of results.

Variable, independent. A variable that is intended or thought to produce a change in the dependent variable. An intervention is a type of independent variable.

Index

Page numbers followed by *f* or *t* indicate figures or tables, respectively.